The International Library

WIT AND ITS RELATION TO
THE UNCONSCIOUS

Founded by C. K. Ogden

The International Library of Psychology

PSYCHOANALYSIS
In 28 Volumes

WIT AND ITS RELATION TO
THE UNCONSCIOUS

SIGMUND FREUD

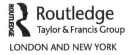

Routledge
Taylor & Francis Group
LONDON AND NEW YORK

First published 1922
by Kegan Paul, Trench, Trubner & Co., Ltd.

Published 2013 by Routledge
2 Park Square, Milton Park, Abingdon, Oxfordshire OX14 4RN
711 Third Avenue, New York, NY 10017, USA

First issued in paperback 2014

Routledge is an imprint of the Taylor & Francis Group, an informa business

© 1922 Sigmund Freud, Translated by A A Brill

All rights reserved. No part of this book may be reprinted or reproduced
or utilized in any form or by any electronic, mechanical, or other means,
now known or hereafter invented, including photocopying
and recording, or in any information storage or retrieval system, without
permission in writing from the publishers.

The publishers have made every effort to contact authors/copyright holders
of the works reprinted in the *International Library of Psychology*.
This has not been possible in every case, however, and we would
welcome correspondence from those individuals/companies
we have been unable to trace.

These reprints are taken from original copies of each book. In many cases
the condition of these originals is not perfect. The publisher has gone to
great lengths to ensure the quality of these reprints, but wishes to point
out that certain characteristics of the original copies will, of necessity, be
apparent in reprints thereof.

British Library Cataloguing in Publication Data
A CIP catalogue record for this book
is available from the British Library

ISBN 978-1-138-87558-6 (pbk)
ISBN 978-0-415-21091-1 (hbk)

Wit and its Relation to the Unconscious
ISBN 0415-21091-7
Psychoanalysis: 28 Volumes
ISBN 0415-21132-8
The International Library of Psychology: 204 Volumes
ISBN 0415-19132-7

TRANSLATOR'S PREFACE

IN 1908 when it was agreed between Professor Freud and myself that I should be his translator, it was decided to render into English first the following five works: *Selected Papers on Hysteria and Psychoneuroses,*[1] *Three Contributions to the Theory of Sex,*[2] *The Interpretation of Dreams,*[3] *Psychopathology of Everyday Life,*[4] and the present volume. These works were selected because they represent the various stages of development of Professor Freud's Psychoanalysis,[5] and also because it was thought that they contain the material which one must master before one is able to judge correctly the author's theories or apply them in practice. This undertaking, which was fraught with many linguistic and other difficulties, has finally been accom-

[1] Monograph Series, Journal of Nervous and Mental Diseases Pub. Co., 2nd Ed., 1912.

[2] Monograph Series, Journal of Nervous and Mental Diseases Pub. Co., 2nd Ed., 1916.

[3] The Macmillan Co., New York, and Allen & Unwin, London.

[4] The Macmillan Co., New York, and T. Fisher Unwin, London.

[5] This expression is used advisedly in order to distinguish it from other methods of "analysis," which Professor Freud fully disavows. Cf. *The History of the Psychoanalytic Movement,* translated by A. A. Brill, *The Psychoanalytic Review,* June-Sept., 1916.

plished with the edition of the present volume, and it is therefore with a sense of great satisfaction that the translator's preface to this work is written. But although the original task is finished the translator's work is only beginning. Psychoanalysis has made enormous strides. On the foundation laid by Professor Freud there developed a literature rich in ideas and content which has revolutionized the science of nervous and mental diseases, and has thrown much light on the subject of dreams, sex, mythology,[1] the history of civilization and racial psychology,[2] philology,[3] æsthetics,[4] child psychology and pedagogics,[5] philology,[6] and mysticism and occultism. With the *Interpretation of Dreams* and *Psychopathology of Everyday Life,* Professor Freud has definitely bridged the gulf between normal and abnormal mental states by demonstrating that dreams and faulty acts like some forms of forgetting, slips of the tongue, slips of reading, writing, etc., are closely allied to psycho-

---

[1] Cf. the works of Freud, Abraham, Rank, and others.

[2] Cf. Freud: *Totem and Taboo,* a translation in preparation, and the works of Jones, Rank and Sachs, Jung, and Storfer.

[3] Cf. Freud, Berny, Rank, and Sachs, and Sperber.

[4] Cf. Freud: *Leonardo da Vinci,* a translation in preparation, and the works of many others.

[5] Cf. v. Hug-Hellmuth: *Aus dem Seelenleben des Kindes,* and the works of Jones, Pfister, and many others.

[6] Cf. the works of Freud, Putnam, Hitschmann, Winterstein, and others.

pathological states and represent the prototypes of such abnormal mental conditions as neurotic symptoms, hallucinations, and deliria. He also shows that all these productions are senseful and purposive, and that their strange and peculiar appearance is due to distortions produced by various psychic processes. These views are confirmed in the present volume, where it is demonstrated that wit, which belongs to æsthetics, is subject to the same laws, shows the same mechanism, and serves the same tendencies as the other psychic productions. With his wonted profundity and ingenuity the author adds the solution of wit to those of the neuroses, dreams, and psychopathological acts.

I take great pleasure in tendering my thanks to Mr. Horatio Winslow, who has read the manuscript and has given me valuable suggestions in the choice of expressions and in the selection of substitutes for those witticisms that could not be translated.

A. A. BRILL.

CONTENTS

A. ANALYSIS OF WIT

B. SYNTHESIS OF WIT

C. THEORIES OF WIT

A. ANALYSIS

WIT AND ITS RELATION TO THE UNCONSCIOUS

I

WHOEVER has had occasion to examine that part of the literature of æsthetics and psychology dealing with the nature and affinities of wit, will, no doubt, concede that our philosophical inquiries have not awarded to wit the important rôle that it plays in our mental life. One can recount only a small number of thinkers who have penetrated at all deeply into the problems of wit. To be sure, among the authors on wit one finds the illustrious names of the poet Jean Paul (Fr. Richter), and of the philosophers Th. Vischer, Kuno Fischer, and Th. Lipps. But even these writers put the subject of wit in the background while their chief interest centers around the more comprehensive and more alluring problems of the comic.

In the main this literature gives the impression that it is altogether impractical to study wit except when treated as a part of the comic.

Presentation of the Subject by Other Authors

According to Th. Lipps (*Komik und Humor,* 1898 [1]) wit is "essentially the subjective side of the comic; i.e., it is that part of the comic which we ourselves create, which colors our conduct as such, and to which our relation is that of Superior Subject, never of Object, certainly not Voluntary Object" (p. 80). The following comment might also be added:—In general we designate as wit "every conscious and clever evocation of the comic, whether the comic element lies in the viewpoint or in the situation itself" (p. 78).

K. Fischer explains the relation between wit and the comic by the aid of caricature, which, according to his exposition, comes midway between the two (*Über den Witz,* 1889). The subject of the comic is the hideous element in any of its manifestations. "Where it is concealed it must be disclosed in the light of the comic view; where it is not at all or but slightly noticeable it must be rendered conspicuous and elucidated in such a manner that it becomes clear and intelligible. Thus arises caricature" (p. 45). "Our entire psychic world, the intellectual realm of our thoughts and concep-

---

[1] *Beiträge zur Aesthetik,* edited by Theodor Lipps and Richard Maria Werner, VI,—a book to which I am indebted for the courage and capacity to undertake this attempt.

tions, does not reveal itself to us on superficial consideration. It cannot be visualized directly either figuratively, or intuitively, moreover it contains inhibitions, weak points, disfigurements, and an abundance of ludicrous and comical contrasts. In order to bring it out and to make it accessible to æsthetic examination, a force is necessary which is capable not only of depicting objects directly, but also of reflecting upon these conceptions and elucidating them— namely, a force capable of clarifying thought. This force is nothing but judgment. The judgment which produces the comic contrast is wit. In caricature wit has played its part unnoticed, but only in judgment does it attain its own individual form and the free domain of its evolution."

As can be seen Lipps assigns the determining factor which classifies wit as part of the comic, to the activity or to the active behavior of the subject, whereas K. Fischer characterizes wit by its relation to its object, in which characterization he accentuates the hidden hideous element in the realm of thought. One cannot put to test the cogency of these definitions of wit; one can, in fact, hardly understand them unless one studies the text from which they were taken. One is thus forced to work his way through the author's descriptions of the comic

in order to learn anything about wit. From
other passages, however, one discovers that the
same authors attribute to wit essential characteristics of general validity in which they disregard its relation to the comic.

K. Fischer's characterization of wit which
seems to be most satisfactory to this author runs
as follows: "Wit is a playful judgment." (p.
51). For an elucidation of this expression we
are referred to the analogy: "How æsthetic
freedom consists in the playful contemplation
of objects " (p. 50). In another place (p. 20)
the æsthetic attitude towards an object is characterized by the condition that we expect nothing from this object—especially no gratification
of our serious needs—but that we content ourselves with the pleasure of contemplating the
same. In contrast to labor the æsthetic attitude
is playful. " It may be that from æsthetic freedom there also results a kind of judgment, freed
from the conventional restrictions and rule of
conduct, which, in view of its genesis, I will
call the playful judgment. This conception contains the first condition and possibly the entire
formula for the solution of our problem. ' Freedom begets wit and wit begets freedom,' says
Jean Paul. Wit is nothing but a free play of
ideas " (p. 24).

Since time immemorial a favorite definition

of wit has been the ability to discover similarities in dissimilarities, i.e., to find hidden similarities. Jean Paul has jocosely expressed this idea by saying that "wit is the disguised priest who unites every couple." Th. Vischer adds the postscript: "He likes best to unite those couples whose marriage the relatives refuse to sanction." Vischer refutes this, however, by remarking that in some witticisms there is no question of comparison or the discovery of similarities. Hence with very little deviation from Jean Paul's definition he defines wit as the skill to combine with surprising quickness many ideas, which through inner content and connections are foreign to one another. K. Fischer then calls attention to the fact that in a large number of these witty judgments one does not find similarities, but contrasts; and Lipps further remarks that these definitions refer to the wit that the humorist possesses and not to the wit that he produces.

Other viewpoints, in some measure connected with one another, which have been mentioned in defining and describing wit are: "the *contrast of ideas*," "*sense in nonsense*," and "*confusion and clearness*."

Definitions like those of Kraepelin lay stress upon the contrast of ideas. Wit is "the voluntary combination or linking of two ideas which in some way are contrasted with each other, usually through the medium of speech association." For a critic like Lipps it would not be difficult to reveal the utter inadequacy of this formula, but he himself does not exclude the element of contrast—he merely assigns it elsewhere. "The contrast remains, but is not formed in a manner to show the ideas connected with the words, rather it shows the contrast or contradiction in the meaning and lack of meaning of the words" (p. 87). Examples show the better understanding of the latter. " A contrast arises first through the fact that we adjudge a. meaning to its words which after all we cannot ascribe to them."

In the further development of this last condition the antithesis of " sense in nonsense " becomes obvious. " What we accept one moment as senseful we later perceive as perfect nonsense. Thereby arises, in this case, the operation of the comic element" (p. 85). " A saying appears witty when we ascribe to it a meaning through psychological necessity and, while so doing, retract it. It may thus have many meanings. We lend a meaning to an expression knowing that logically it does not belong to it. We find in it a truth, however, which later we fail to find because it is foreign to our laws of experience or usual modes of thinking. We endow it with a logical or practical inference which transcends its true content, only to contradict this inference as soon as we finally grasp the nature of the expression itself. The psychological process evoked in us by the witty expression which gives rise to the sense of the comic depends in every case on the immediate transition from the borrowed feeling of truth and conviction to the impression or consciousness of relative nullity."

As impressive as this exposition sounds one cannot refrain from questioning whether the contrast between the senseful and senseless upon which the comic depends does not also contribute to the definition of wit in so far as it is distinguished from the comic. Also the factor of " confusion and clearness " leads one deeply into the problem of the relation of wit to the comic. Kant, speaking of the comic element in general, states that one of its remarkable attributes is the fact that it can delude us for a moment only. Heymans (*Zeitschr. f. Psychologie,* XI, 1896) explains how the mechanism of wit is produced through the succession of confusion and clearness. He illustrates his meaning by an excellent witticism from Heine, who causes one of his figures, the poor lottery agent, Hirsch-Hyacinth, to boast that the great Baron Rothschild treated him as an equal or quite FAMILLIONAIRE. Here the word which acts as the carrier of the

witticism appears in tne first place simply as a
faulty word-formation, as something incomprehensible, inconceivable, and enigmatic. It is for
these reasons that it is confusing. The comic
element results from the solution of the enigma
and from the understanding of the word. Lipps
adds that the first stage of enlightenment, showing that the confusing word means this or that, is
followed by a second stage in which one perceives
that this nonsensical word has first deluded us
and then given us the true meaning. Only this
second enlightenment, the realization that it is
all due to a word that is meaningless in ordinary
usage—this reduction to nothingness produces
the comic effect (p. 95).

Whether or not either the one or the other
of these two conceptions may seem more clear
we are brought nearer to a definite insight
through the discussion of the processes of confusion and enlightenment. If the comic effect of
Heine's *famillionaire* depends upon the solution
of the seemingly senseless word, then the wit
would have to be attributed to the formation of
this word and to the character of the word so
formed.

In addition to the associations of the viewpoints just discussed there is another characteristic of wit which is recognized as peculiar to it
by all authors. " Brevity alone is the body and

soul of wit," declares Jean Paul (*Vorschule der Aesthetik,* I, 45), and modifies it with a speech of the old tongue-wagger, Polonius, from Shakespeare's *Hamlet* (Act II, Scene 2):

" Therefore, since brevity is the soul of wit,
  And tediousness the limbs and outward flourishes,
  I will be brief."

Lipps's description (p. 90) of the brevity of wit is also significant. He states that wit says what it does say, not always in few, but always in too few words; that is: " It expresses itself in words that will not stand the test of strict logic or of the ordinary mode of thought and expression. In fine it can express itself by leaving the thing unsaid."

That " wit must unearth something hidden and concealed "—to quote K. Fischer (p. 51)—we have already been taught from the grouping of wit with caricature. I re-emphasize this determinant because it also has more to do with the nature of wit than with its relation to the comic.

I am well aware that the foregoing scanty quotations from the works of the authors on wit cannot do justice to the excellence of these works. In view of the difficulties that confront one in reproducing clearly such complicated and such delicately shaded streams of thought I cannot

spare inquiring minds the trouble of searching
for the desired information in the original
sources. However, I do not know whether they
will return fully satisfied. For the criteria and
attributes of wit mentioned by these authors,
such as—activity, the relation of the content of
wit to our thoughts, the character of the playful
judgment, the union of dissimilarities, contrasting ideas, " sense in nonsense," the succession of
confusion and clearness, the sudden emergence
of the hidden, and the peculiar brevity of wit,
seem to us, at first glance, so very pertinent and
so easily demonstrable by examples that we cannot succumb to the danger of underestimating
the value of such ideas. But they are only dis-
jointed fragments which we should like to see
welded into an organic whole. In the end they
contribute no more to the knowledge of wit than
a number of anecdotes teach us of the true characteristics of a personality whose biography interests us. We do not at all understand the connection that is supposed to exist between the individual conditions; for instance, what the brevity of wit may have to do with that side of wit
exhibited in the playful judgment; besides we do
not know whether wit must satisfy all or only
some of these conditions in order to form real
wit; which of them may be replaced and which
ones are indispensable. We should also like a

grouping and classification of wit in respect to its essential attributes. The classification as given by the authors is based, on the one hand, on the technical means, and on the other hand, on the utilization of wit in speech (sound-wit, play on words, the wit of caricature, characterization wit, and witty repartee).

Accordingly we should not find ourselves in a dilemma when it comes to pointing out goals for a further effort to explain wit. In order to look forward to success we must either introduce new viewpoints into the work, or try to penetrate further by concentrating our attention or by broadening the scope of our interest. We can prescribe for ourselves the task of at least not permitting any lack along the latter lines. To be sure, it is rather remarkable how few examples of recognized witticisms suffice the authors for their investigations and how each one accepts the ones used by his predecessors. We need not shirk the responsibility of analyzing the same examples which have already served the classical authors, but we contemplate new material besides to lay a broader foundation for our deductions. It is quite natural that we should select such examples of wit as objects for our investigation as have produced the deepest impression upon our own lives and which have caused us the greatest amount of laughter.

Some may inquire whether the subject of wit is worthy of such effort. In my opinion there is no doubt about it, for even if I disregard the personal motives to be revealed during the development of this theme (the motives which drove me to gain an insight into the problem of wit), I can refer to the fact that there is an intimate connection between all psychic occurrences; a connection which promises to furnish a psychological insight into a sphere which, although remote, will nevertheless be of considerable value to the other spheres. One may also be reminded what a peculiar, overwhelmingly fascinating charm wit offers in our society. A new joke operates almost as an event of universal interest. It is passed on from one person to another just like the news of the latest conquest. Even prominent men who consider it worth while relating how they attained fame, what cities and countries they have seen, and with what celebrated persons they have consorted, do not disdain to dwell in their autobiographies upon this and that excellent joke which they have heard.[1]

[1] J. V. Falke: *Lebenserinnerungen*, 1897.

II

WE follow the beckoning of chance and take up as our first example of wit one which has already come to our notice in the previous chapter.

In that part of the *Reisebilder* entitled " Die Bäder von Lucca," Heine introduces the precious character, Hirsch-Hyacinth, the Hamburg lottery agent and curer of corns, who, boasting to the poet of his relationship with the rich Baron Rothschild, ends thus: " And as true as I pray that the Lord may grant me all good things I sat next to Solomon Rothschild, who treated me just as if I were his equal, quite *famillionaire.*"

It is by means of this excellent and very funny example that Heymans and Lipps have illustrated the origin of the comic effect of wit from the succession of " confusion and clearness." However, we shall pass over this question and put to ourselves the following inquiry: What is it that causes the speech of Hirsch-Hyacinth to become witty? It can be only one of two things; either it is the thought expressed in the sentence which carries in itself the character of the witticism; or the witticism adheres to the mode of ex-

15

pression which clothes the thought. On whichever side the nature of the wit may lie, there we shall follow it farther and endeavor to elucidate it.

In general a thought may be expressed in different forms of speech—that is, in different words—which may repeat it in its original accuracy. In the speech of Hirsch-Hyacinth we have before us a definite form of thought expressed which seems to us especially peculiar and not very readily comprehensible. Let us attempt to express as exactly as is possible the same thought in other words. Lipps, indeed, has already done this and has thus, to some degree, elucidated the meaning of the poet. He says (p. 87), "We understand that Heine wishes to say that the reception was on a familiar basis, that is, that it was of the friendly sort." We change nothing in the sense when we assume a different interpretation which perhaps fits better into the speech of Hirsch-Hyacinth: "Rothschild treated me quite as his equal, in a very *familiar* way; that is, as far as this can be done by a *millionaire.*" We would only add, "The condescension of a rich man always carries something embarrassing for the one experiencing it." [1]

---

[1] Since this joke will occupy us again and we do not wish to disturb the discussion following here, we shall find occasion later to point out a correction in Lipps's given interpretation which follows our own.

Whether we shall remain content with this or with another equivalent formulation of the thought, we can see that the question which we have put to ourselves is already answered. The character of the wit in this example does not adhere to the thought. It is a correct and ingenious remark that Heine puts into the mouth of Hirsch-Hyacinth—a remark of indubitable bitterness, as is easily understood in the case of the poor man confronted with so much wealth; but we should not care to call it witty. Now if any one who cannot forget the poet's meaning in the interpretation should insist that the thought in itself is also witty, we can refer him to the definite fact that the witty character is lost in the interpretation. It is true that Hirsch-Hyacinth's speech made us laugh loudly, but though Lipps's or our own accurate rendering may please us and cause us to reflect, yet it cannot make us laugh.

But if the witty character of our example does not belong to the thought, then it must be sought for in the form of expression in the wording. We have only to study the peculiarity of this mode of expression to realize what one may term word- or form-technique. Also we may discover the things that are intimately related to the very nature of wit, since the character as well as the effect of wit disappears when one set of expres-

sions is changed for others. At all events we
are in full accord with our authors when we put
so much value upon the verbal form of the wit.
Thus K. Fischer (p. 72) says: " It is, in the first
place, the naked form which is responsible for
the perception of wit, and one is reminded of a
saying of Jean Paul's which affirms and proves
this nature of wit in the same expression. ' Thus
the mere position conquers, be it that of warriors
or of sentences.' "

Formation of Mixed Words

Now wherein lies the "'technique" of this
wit? What has occurred to the thought, in our
own conception, that it became changed into wit
and caused us to laugh heartily? The comparison of our conception with the text of the poet
teaches us that two processes took place. In the
first place there occurred an important abbreviation. In order to express fully the thought contained in the witticism we had to append to the
words "Rothschild treated me just as an equal,
on a familiar basis," an additional sentence
which in its briefest form reads: i.e., so far as
a millionaire can do this. Even then we feel the
necessity of an additional explanatory sentence.[1]
The poet expresses it in terser terms as follows:
"Rothschild treated me just like an equal,

---

[1] The same holds true for Lipps's interpretation.

quite *famillionaire."*   The entire restriction, which the second sentence imposes on the first thus verifying the familiar treatment, has been lost in the jest.   But it has not been so entirely lost as not to leave a substitute from which it can be reconstructed.   A second change has also taken place.   The word " familiar " in the wit- less expression of the thought has been trans- formed into *" famillionaire "* in the text of the wit, and there is no doubt that the witty char- acter and ludicrous effect of the joke depends directly upon this word-formation.   The newly formed word is identical in its first part with the word " familiar " of the first sentence, and its terminal syllables correspond to the word " millionaire " of the second sentence.   In this manner it puts us in a position to conjecture the second sentence which was omitted in the text of the wit.   It may be described as a composite of two constituents " familiar " and " million- aire," and one is tempted to depict its origin from the two words graphically.

FAMIL I   A R
MILLIONAIRE
———————————————
FAMILLIONAIRE

The process, then, which has carried the thought into the witticism can be represented in the following manner, which, although at first rather fantastic, nevertheless furnishes exactly the actual existing result: "Rothschild treated me quite familiarly, i.e., as well as a millionaire can do that sort of thing."

Now imagine that a compressing force is acting upon these sentences and assume that for some reason or other the second sentence is of lesser resistance. It is accordingly forced toward the vanishing point, but its important component, the word "millionaire," which strives against the compressing power, is pushed, as it were, into the first sentence and becomes fused with the very similar element, the word "familiar" of this sentence. It is just this possibility, provided by chance to save the essential part of the second sentence, which favors the disappearance of the other less important components. The jest then takes shape in this manner: "Rothschild treated me in a very famillionaire way."
(mili) (aire)

Apart from such a compressing force, which is really unknown to us, we may describe the origin of the wit-formation, that is, the technique of the wit in this case, as a *condensation with substitutive formation*. In our example the substitutive formation consists in the formation of a mixed word. This fused word "famillionaire," incomprehensible in itself but instantly understood in its context and recognized as senseful, is now the carrier of the mirth-provoking stimulus of the jest, whose mechanism, to be sure, is in no way clearer to us through the discovery of the technique. To what extent can a linguistic process of condensation with substitutive formation produce pleasure through a fused word and force us to laugh? We make note of the fact that this is a different problem, the treatment of which we can postpone until we shall find access to it later. For the present we shall continue to busy ourselves with the technique of wit.

Our expectation that the technique of wit cannot be considered an indifferent factor in the examination of the nature of wit prompts us to inquire next whether there are other examples of wit formed like Heine's "famillionaire." Not many of these exist, but enough to constitute a small group which may be characterized as the blend-word formations or fusions. Heine himself has produced a second witticism from the word "millionaire" by copying himself, as it were, when he speaks of a "millionarr" (*Ideen,* Chap. XIV). This is a visible condensation of "millionaire" and "narr" (fool) and, like the first example, expresses a suppressed by-thought. Other examples of a similar nature are as follows.

During the war between Turkey and the Balkan States, in 1912, *Punch* depicted the part played by Rumania by representing the latter as a highwayman holding up the members of the Balkan alliance. The picture was entitled: *Kleptorumania.* Here the word is a fusion of Kleptomania and Rumania and may be represented as follows:

KLEPTOMANIA

RUMANIA

KLEPTORUMANIA

A naughty jest of Europe has rebaptized a former potentate, Leopold, into *Cleopold* because of his relation to a lady surnamed Cleo. This is a clear form of condensation which by the addition of a single letter forever vividly preserves a scandalous allusion.

In an excellent chapter on this same theme Brill gives the following example.[1]

" De Quincey once remarked that old persons are apt to fall into ' anecdotage.' " The word *Anecdotage,* though in itself incomprehensible, can be readily analyzed to show its original full sense; and on analysis we find that it is made up of two words, *anecdote* and *dotage.* That is, in-

---

[1] *Psychanalysis:* Its Theories and Application, 2nd Ed., p. 331.

stead of saying that old persons are apt to fall
into dotage and that old persons are fond of telling anecdotes, De Quincey fuses the two words
into a neologism, *anecdotage,* and thus simultaneously expresses both ideas.   The technique,
therefore, lies in the fusion of the two words.
Such a fusion of words is called condensation.
Condensation is a substitutive formation, i.e., instead of *anecdote* and *dotage* we have *anecdotage.*

" In a short story which I have recently read,
one of the characters, a ' sport,' speaks of the
Christmas season as the *alcoholidays.* By reduction it can be easily seen that we have here a com-
pound word, a combination of *alcohol* and *holidays* which can be graphically represented as
follows:

alco H O L

H O L i d a y s

ALCOHOLIDAYS

" Here the condensation expresses the idea
that holidays are conducive to alcoholic indulgence.   In other words, we have here a fused
word, which, though strange in appearance, can
be easily understood in its proper context. The
witticism may be described as a condensation
with substitution.

" The same mechanism is found in the following: A dramatic critic, summarizing three para-

graphs to the effect that most plays now produced in New York City are violently emotional
and hysterical, remarks: ' Thespis has taken up
his home in Dramatteawan.' The last word is
a condensation of *drama* and *Matteawan*. The
substitution not only expressed the critic's idea
that most of the plays at present produced in
New York are violent, emotional and hysterical,
that is insane, but it also contains a clever allusion to the nature of the problem presented by
most of these plays. Matteawan is a state hospi-
tal for criminal insane. Most of the plays are
not only insane, but also criminal since they treat
of murders, divorces, robberies, scandals, etc."

When Flaubert published his famous romance
Salammbo, which treats of life in ancient Car-
thage, it was scoffingly referred to by Sainte-
Beuve as *Carthaginoiserie* on account of its
tedious detailed descriptions.

Carthaginoiserie
chinoiserie

During a conversation with a lady I unintentionally furnished the material for a jest. I
spoke to her about the great merits of an investi-
gator whom I considered unjustly ignored. She
remarked, " But the man really deserves a monument." " Perhaps he will get one some day," I
answered, " but at the moment his success is

very limited." " Monument " and " moment
are contrasts. The lady then united these contrasts and said: " Well, let us wish him a *monu-
mentary* success."

If at this stage the reader should become
displeased with a viewpoint which threatens to
destroy his pleasure in wit without explaining
the source of this pleasure I must beg him to
be patient for a while, because we are now confronted with the technique of wit, the examination of which promises many revelations if
only we enter into it far enough. Besides the
analysis of the examples thus far cited, which
show simply a process of condensation, there
are others in which the changed expressions
manifest themselves in other ways.

Condensation with Modification and Substitution

The following witticisms of Mr. N. will serve
as illustrations.

" I was driving with him tête-à-bête." Nothing is simpler than the reduction of this jest.
Evidently it can only mean: I was driving
tête-à-tête with Mr. X. and X. is a stupid ass
(beast).

Neither of these two sentences is witty nor
is there any wit if one combines them into this
one: " I was out driving tête-à-tête with that
stupid ass (beast)." The wit appears when

the words " stupid ass " are omitted and when, as a substitute for them, the first " t " of the second " tête " is changed to " b." This slight modification brings back to expression the suppressed " bête." The technique of this group of witticisms may be described as " condensation with a slight modification." And it would seem that the more insignificant the substitutive modification, the better is the wit.

Quite similar, although not without its complications, is the technique of another form of witticism. During a discussion about a person in whom there was something to praise and much to criticise, N. remarked: " Yes, vanity is one of his four heels of Achilles." [1] This modification consists in the fact that instead of the one vulnerable heel which was attributed to Achilles we have here four heels. Four heels means four feet and that number is only found on animals. The two thoughts condensed in the witticism are as follows: Except for his vanity he is an admirable fellow; still I do not care for him, for he is more of an animal than a human being.[2]

---

[1] This same witticism was supposed to have been coined before by Heine concerning Alfred de Musset.

[2] One of the complications involved in the technique of this example lies in the fact that the modification through which the omitted abuse is substituted is to be taken as an allusion to the latter, for it leads to it only through a process of deduction.

A similar but simpler joke I heard *statu nascendi* in a family circle. One of two brothers who were attending college was an excellent scholar while the other was only an average student. It so happened that the model boy had a setback in school. The mother discussed this matter and expressed her fear lest this event be the beginning of a lasting deterioration. The boy who until then had been overshadowed by his brother willingly grasped this opportunity to remark: " Yes, Carl is going backward on all-fours."

Here the modification consists in a small addition as an assurance that in his judgment his brother is going backward. This modification represents and takes the place of a passionate plea for his own cause which may be expressed as follows: After all, you must not think that he is so much cleverer than I am simply because he has more success in school. He is really a stupid ass, i.e., much more stupid than I am.

A good illustration of condensation with slight modification is furnished by a well-known witty jest of Mr. N., who remarked about a character in public life that he had a " *great future behind him.*" The butt of this joke was a young man whose ancestry, rearing, and personal qualities seemed to destine him for the leadership of a great party and the attainment of political power at its head. But times changed, the party became politically incompetent, and it could readily be foreseen that the man who was predestined to become its leader would come to nothing. The briefest reduction of the meaning by which one could replace this joke would be: The man has had a great future before him, but that is now past. Instead of " has had " and the appended afterthought there is a small change in the main sentence in which " before " is replaced by its opposite " behind." [1]

Mr. N. made use of almost the same modification in the case of the nobleman who was appointed minister of agriculture for no other reason than that he was interested in agriculture. Public opinion had an opportunity to find out that he was the most incompetent man who had ever been intrusted with this office. When, however, he had relinquished his portfolio and had withdrawn to his agricultural pursuits Mr. N. said of him: " *Like Cincinnatus of Old he has returned to his place in front of the plough.*"

---

[1] Another factor which I shall mention later on is also effective in the technique of this witticism. It has to do with the inner character of the modification (representation through the opposite—contradiction). The technique of wit does not hesitate to make use simultaneously of several means, with which, however, we can only become acquainted in their sequential order.

That Roman, who was likewise called to his office from his farm, returned to his place behind the plough. In those days, just as in the present time, in front of the plough walked—the ox.

We could easily increase these examples by many others, but I am of the opinion that we are in need of no more cases in order to grasp thoroughly the character of the technique of this second group—condensation with modification. If we now compare the second group with the first, the technique of which consisted in condensation with a mixed word-formation, we readily see that the differences are not vital and that the lines of demarcation are indistinct. The mixed word-formation, like the modification, became subordinated to the idea of substitutive formation, and if we desire we can also describe the mixed word-formation as a modification of the parent word through the second elements.

We may make our first pause here and ask ourselves with what known factor in the literature of wit our first result, either in whole or in part, coincides. It obviously agrees with the factor of brevity which Jean Paul calls the soul of wit (*supra,* p. 11). But brevity alone is not wit or every laconism would be witty. The brevity of wit must be of a special kind. We

recall that Lipps has attempted to describe
more fully the peculiarity of the brevity of
wit (*v. s.*, p. 11). Here our investigation started
and demonstrated that the brevity of wit is
often the result of a special process which has
left a second trace—the substitutive formation—
in the wording of the wit. By applying the
process of reduction, which aims to cause a
retrogression in the peculiar process of condensation, we find also that wit depends only
upon the verbal expression which was produced
by the process of condensation. Naturally our
entire interest now centers upon this peculiar
and hitherto almost neglected mechanism.
Furthermore, we cannot yet comprehend how
it can give origin to all that is valuable in wit;
namely, the resultant pleasure.

Condensation in Dreams

Have processes similar to those here described as the technique of wit already been
noted in another sphere of our psychic life?
To be sure, in one apparently remote sphere.
In 1900 I published a book which, as indicated
by its title (*The Interpretation of Dreams* [1]),
makes the attempt to explain the riddle of the
dream and to trace the dream to normal psychic

[1] Translation of 4th Ed. by A. A. Brill, the Macmillan Co.,
New York, and Allen & Unwin, London.

operations. I had occasion to contrast there the manifest and often peculiar dream-content with the latent but altogether real thoughts of the dream from which it originated, and I took up the investigation of the processes which make the dream from the latent dream-thought. I also investigated the psychological forces which participated in this transposition. The sum of the transforming processes I designated as the dream-work and, as a part of this dream-work, I described the process of condensation. This process has a striking similarity to the technique of wit and, like the latter, it leads to abbreviations and brings about substitutive formations of like character.

From recollections of his own dreams the reader will be familiar with the compositions of persons and objects that appear in them; indeed, the dream makes similar compositions of words which can then be reduced by analysis (e.g., Autodidasker—Autodidakt and Lasker [1]). On other occasions and even much more frequently, the condensation work of the dream produces no compositions, but pictures which closely resemble an object or person up to a certain addition or variation which comes from another source, like the modifications in the witticisms of Mr. N. We cannot doubt that

[1] *The Interpretation of Dreams,* p. 280.

in this case, as in the other, we deal with a
similar psychic process which is recognizable by
identical results. Such a far-reaching analogy
between wit-technique and dream-work will
surely arouse our interest in the former and
stimulate our expectation of finding some explanation of wit from a comparison with the
dream. We forbear, however, to enter upon
this work by bearing in mind that we have investigated the technique of wit in only a very
small number of witty jests, so that we cannot
be certain that the analogy, the workings of
which we wish to explore, will hold good.
Hence we turn away from the comparison with
the dream and again take up the technique of
wit, leaving, however, at this place of our investigation a visible thread, as it were, which
later we shall take up again.

Wit Formed by Word-division

The next point we shall discuss is whether the
process of condensation with substitutive formation is demonstrable in all witticisms so that
it may be designated as a universal character of
the technique of wit. I recall a joke which has
clung to my mind through certain peculiar circumstances. One of the great teachers of my
youth, whom we considered unable to appreciate

a joke—he had never told us a single joke of his own—came into the Institute laughing. With an unwonted readiness he explained the cause of his good humor. " I have read an excellent joke," he said. *" A young man who claimed to be a relative of the great J. J. Rousseau, and who bore his name, was introduced into a Parisian drawing-room. It should be added that he was decidedly red-headed. He behaved in such an awkward manner that the hostess ventured this criticism to the gentleman who had introduced him—' Vous m'avez fait connaître un jeune homme roux et sot, mais non pas un Rousseau.' "*

At this point our teacher started to laugh again. According to the nomenclature of our authors this is sound-wit and a poor kind at that, since it plays with a proper name.

But what is the technique of this wit? It is quite clear that the character which we had perhaps hoped to demonstrate universally leaves us in the lurch in the first new example. Here there is no omission and scarcely an abbreviation. In the witticism the lady expresses almost everything that we can ascribe to the thoughts. " You have made me look forward to meeting a relative of J. J. Rousseau. I expected that he was perhaps even mentally related to him. Imagine my surprise to find this red-haired foolish boy, a *roux et sot.*" To be sure, I was able to add and insert something, but this attempt at reduction does not annul the wit. It remains fixed and attached to the sound similarity of Rousseau. This proves that con-

$$\frac{\text{con-}}{\text{roux sot}}$$

densation with substitution plays no part in the production of this witticism.

With what else do we have to deal? New attempts at reduction taught me that the joke will persistently continue until the name Rousseau is replaced by another. If, e.g., I substitute the name Racine for it I find that although the lady's criticism is just as feasible as before it immediately loses every trace of wit. Now I know where I can look for the technique of this joke although I still hesitate to formulate it. I shall make the following attempt: The technique of the witticism lies in the fact that one and the same word—the name—is used in a twofold application, once as a whole and once divided into its syllables like a charade.

I can mention a few examples of identical technique. A witticism of this sort was utilized by an Italian lady to avenge a tactless remark made to her by the first Napoleon. Pointing to her compatriots at a court ball he said: "*Tutti gli Italian danzano si male*" (all Italians dance so badly). To which she quickly replied: "*Non tutti, ma buona parte*" (Not all, but a great many)—Buona parte.[1] Brill

Buonaparte.

reports still another example in which the wit depends on the twofold application of a name: "*Hood once remarked that he had to be a lively Hood for a livelihood.*"[2]

At one time when Antigone was produced in Berlin a critic found that the presentation entirely lacked the character of antiquity. The wits of Berlin incorporated this criticism in the following manner: "*Antique? Oh, nay*" (Th. Vischer and K. Fischer).

Manifold Application of the Same Material

In these examples, which will suffice for this species of wit, the technique is the same. A name is made use of twice; first, as a whole, and then divided into its syllables—and in their divided state the syllables yield a different meaning.[3] The manifold application of the same word, once as a whole and then as the component syllables into which it divides itself, was the first case that came to our attention in which technique deviated from that of con-

[1] Cited by Brill: *Psychanalysis*, p. 335.
[2] l. c., p. 334.
[3] The excellence of these jokes depends upon the fact that they, at the same time, present another technical means of a much higher order.

densation. Upon brief reflection, however, we must divine from the abundance of examples that come to us that the newly discovered technique can hardly be limited to this single means. Obviously there are any number of hitherto unobserved possibilities for one to utilize the same word or the same material of words in manifold application *in one sentence*. May not all these possibilities furnish technical means for wit? It would seem so, judging by the following examples.

"*Two witty statesmen, X and Y, met at a dinner. X, acting as toastmaster, introduced Y as follows: 'My friend, Y, is a very wonderful man. All you have to do is to open his mouth, put in a dinner, and a speech appears, etc.' Responding to the speaker, Y said: 'My friend, the toastmaster, told you what a wonderful man I am, that all you have to do is to open my mouth, put in a dinner, and a speech appears. Now let me tell you what a wonderful man he is. All you have to do is open anybody's mouth, put in his speech, and the dinner appears.'*" [1]

In examples of this sort, one can use the same material of words and simply change slightly their order. The slighter the change, the more one gets the impression that differ-

---

[1] Given by Translator.

ent sense was expressed with the same words, the better is the technical means of wit. And how simple are the means of its production! *"Put in a dinner and a speech appears—put in a speech and a dinner appears."* This is really nothing but an exchange of places of these two phrases whereby what was said of Y becomes differentiated from what is said of X. To be sure, this is not the whole technique of the joke.[1]

Great latitude is afforded the technique of wit if one so extends the *"manifold application of the same material"* that the word—or the words—upon which the wit depends may be used first unchanged and then with a slight modification. An example is another joke of Mr. N. He heard a gentleman, who himself was born a Jew, utter a malicious statement about Jewish character. "Mr. Councilor," said he, "I am familiar with your *antesemitism,* but your *antisemitism* is new to me."

Here only one single letter is changed, the modification of which could hardly be noticed in careless pronunciation. This example reminds one of the other modification jokes of

---

[1] This resembles an excellent joke of Oliver Wendell Holmes cited by Brill: "Put not your trust in money, but put your money in trust." A contradiction is here announced which does not appear. At all events it is a good example of the untranslatableness of the witticisms of such technique.

Mr. N., but it differs from them in lacking the condensation. Everything that was to be said has been told in the joke. " I know that you yourself were formerly a Jew, therefore I am surprised that you should rail against the Jew."

An excellent example of such wit modification is also the familiar exclamation: " *Traduttore—Traditore.*" [1]

The similarity between the two words, almost approaching identity, results in a very impressive representation of the inevitability by which a translator becomes a transgressor—in the eyes of the author.

The manifoldness of slight modifications possible in these jokes is so great that none is quite similar to the other. Here is a joke which is supposed to have arisen at an examination for the degree of law. The candidate was translating a passage from the Corpus juris, "*Labeo ait.*" " ' I fall (fail),' says he," volunteered the candidate. " ' You fall (fail),' says I," replied the examiner and the examination ended. Whoever mistakes the name of the celebrated Jurist for a word to which he attaches a false meaning certainly deserves nothing better. But the technique of the witticism lies in the fact

---

[1] Brill cites a very analogous modification wit: *Amantes—Amentes* (lovers—lunatics).

that the examiner used almost the same words in punishing the applicant which the latter used to prove his ignorance. Besides, the joke is an example of repartee whose technique, as we shall see, is closely allied to the one just mentioned.

Words are plastic and may be moulded into almost any shape. There are some words which have lost their true original meaning in certain usages which they still enjoy in other applications. In one of Lichtenberg's jokes just those conditions have been sought for in which the nuances of the wordings have removed their basic meaning.

" How goes it? " asked the blind of the lame one. " As you see," replied the lame one to the blind.

Language is replete with words which taken in one sense are full of meaning and in another are colorless. There may be two different derivatives from the same root, one of which may develop into a word with a full meaning while the other may become a colorless suffix or prefix, and yet both may have the same sound. The similarity of sound between a word having full meaning and one whose meaning is colorless may also be accidental. In both cases the technique of wit can make use of such relationship of the speech material. The following examples illustrate some of these points.

"*Do you call a man kind who remits nothing to his family while away?*" asked an actor. "*Call that kindness?*" "*Yes, unremitting kindness,*" was the reply of Douglas Jerrold. The wit here depends on the first syllable *un* of the word *unremitting*. *Un* is usually a prefix denoting "not," but by adding it to "remitting" a new relationship is unexpectedly established which changes the meaning of the context. "*An undertaker is one who always carries out what he undertakes.*" The striking character upon which the wit here depends is the manifold application of the words *undertaker* and *carry out*. Undertaker commonly denotes one who manages funerals. Only when taken in this sense and using the words *carry out* literally is the sentence witty. The wit lies in the manifold application of the same words.

Double Meaning and Play on Words

If we delve more deeply into the variety of "manifold application" of the same word we suddenly notice that we are confronted with forms of "double meaning" or "plays on words" which have been known a long time and which are universally acknowledged as belonging to the technique of wit. Then why have we bothered our brains about discovering something new when we could just as well have gleaned it from the most superficial treatise on wit? We can say in self-defense only that we are presenting another side of the same phenomena of verbal expressions. What the authors call the "playful" character of wit we treat from the point of view of "manifold application."

Further examples of manifold application which may also be designated under a new and third group, the class of double meaning, may be divided into subdivisions. These, to be sure, are not essentially differentiated from one another any more than the whole third group from the second. In the first place we have:

(a) Cases of double meaning of a name and its verbal significance: e.g., "*Discharge thyself of our company, Pistol*" (*Henry IV*, Act II). "*For Suffolk's duke may he suffocate*" (*Henry IV*, Act I). Heine says, "*Here in Hamburg rules not the rascally Macbeth, but Banko* (Banquo)."

In those cases where the unchanged name cannot be used,—one might say "misused,"—one can get a double meaning by means of familiar slight modifications: "*Whu have the*

French rejected Lohengrin?" was a question asked some time ago. The answer was, "*On Elsa's* (Alsace) *account.*"

(b) Cases where a double meaning is obtained by using a word which has both a verbal and metaphoric sense furnish an abundant source for the technique of wit. A medical colleague, who was well known for his wit, once said to Arthur Schnitzler, the writer: "*I am not at all surprised that you became a great poet. Your father had already held up the mirror to his contemporaries.*" The mirror used by the father of the writer, the famous Dr. Schnitzler, was the laryngoscope. According to the well-known quotation from *Hamlet* (Act III, Scene 2), the object of the play as well as the writer who creates it is to "hold, as 't were, the mirror up to nature; to show virtue her own feature, scorn her own image, and the very age and body of the time his form and pressure."

(c) Cases of actual double meaning or play on words—the ideal case, as it were, of manifold application. Here no violence is done to the word. It is not torn into syllables. It need not undergo any modifications. It need not exchange its own particular sphere, say as a proper name, for another. Thanks to certain circumstances it can express two meanings just

as it stands in the structure of the sentence.
Many examples are at our disposal.

One of the first royal acts of the last Napoleon was, as is well known, the confiscation
of the estates belonging to the House of Or-
leans. *"C'est le premier vol de l'aigle"* was
an excellent play on words current at that time.
"Vol" means both flight and theft. Louis XV
wished to test the wit of one of his courtiers
whose talent in that direction he had heard
about. He seized his first opportunity to command the cavalier to concoct a joke at his
(the king's) expense. He wanted to be the
"subject" of the witticism. The courtier answered him with the clever *bonmot*, *"Le roi
n'est pas sujet."* "Subject" also means "vas-
sal." (Taken from K. Fischer.)

*A physician, leaving the sick-bed of a wife,
whose husband accompanied him, exclaimed
doubtfully: "I do not like her looks." "I
have not liked her looks for a long time," was
the quick rejoinder of the husband.* The
physician, of course, referred to the condition
of the wife, but he expressed his apprehension
about the patient in such words as to afford
the husband the means of utilizing them to
assert his conjugal aversion. Concerning a
satirical comedy Heine remarked: *"This satire
would not have been so biting had the author*

of it had more to bite." This jest is a better example of metaphoric and common double meaning than of real play upon words, but at present we are not concerned about such strict lines of demarcation. *Charles Matthews, the elder, one of England's greatest actors, was asked what he was going to do with his son* (the young man was destined for architecture). *" Why,"* answered the comedian, *" he is going to draw houses like his father."* Foote *once asked a man why he forever sang one tune.* *" Because it haunts me,"* replied the man. *" No wonder,"* said Foote, *" you are continually murdering it."* Said the Dyspeptic Philosopher: *" One swallow doesn't make a summer, nor quench the thirst."*

A gentleman had shown much ingenuity in evading a notorious borrower whom he had sent away many times with the request to call when he was " in." One day, however, the borrower eluded the servant at the door and cornered his victim.

" Ah," said the host, seeing there was no way out of it, *" at last I am in."*

" No," returned the borrower in anticipation, *"at last I am in and you are out."*

Heine said in the *Harzreise:* *" I cannot recall at the moment the names of all the students, and among the professors there are some who have no name as yet."*

Dr. Johnson said of the University of St. Andrews in Scotland, which was poor in purse, but prolific in the distribution of its degrees: *" Let it persevere in its present plan and it may become rich by degrees."* Here the wit depends more on the manifold application than on the play on words.

The keen-witted writer, Horatio Winslow, sums up the only too-familiar history of some American families as follows:

A TALE OF TWO AMERICAN GENERATIONS
Gold Mine
Gold Spoon
Gold Cure

The last couplet, gold cure, refers to the familiar cure for alcoholism. This wit is an excellent example of unification—everything is, as it were, of gold. The manifold meanings of the adjective which do not very strikingly contrast with one another make possible this " manifold application."

Ambiguity

Another play on words will facilitate the transition to a new subdivision of the technique of double meaning. The witty colleague who was responsible for the joke mentioned on page 42 is likewise responsible for this joke, current during the trial of Dreyfus:

"*This girl reminds me of Dreyfus. The army does not believe in her innocence.*"

The word innocence, whose double meaning furnishes the basis of the witticism, has in one connection the customary meaning which is the opposite of guilt or transgression, while in the other connection it has a sexual sense, the opposite of which is sexual experience. There are very many such examples of double meaning and in each one the point of the joke refers especially to a sexual sense. The group could be designated as "ambiguous." *A good example to illustrate this is the story told of a wealthy but elderly gentleman who showed his devotion to a young actress by many lavish gifts. Being a respectable girl she took the first opportunity to discourage his attentions by telling him that her heart was already given to another man. "I never aspired as high as that," was his polite answer.*

If one compares this example of double-meaning-with-ambiguity with other examples one cannot help noticing a difference which is not altogether inconsequential to the technique. In the joke about "innocence" one meaning of the word is just as good for our understanding of it as the other. One can really not decide whether the sexual or non-sexual significance of the word is more applicable and more familiar. But it is different with the other example mentioned. Here the final sense of the words, "I never aspired as high as that," is by far more obtrusive and covers and conceals, as it were, the sexual sense which could easily escape the unsuspecting person. In sharp contrast to this let us examine another example of double meaning in which there is no attempt made to veil its sexual significance—e.g., Heine's characterization of a complaisant lady: *"She could pass (abschlagen) nothing except her water."* It sounds like an obscene joke and the wit in it is scarcely noticed.[1] But the peculiarity that both senses of the double meaning are not equally manifested can occur also in witticisms without sexual reference providing that one sense is more common or that it is preferred on account of its connection with the other parts of the sentence (e.g., *c'est le premier vol de l'aigle*). All these examples I propose to call double meaning with allusion.

---

[1] Compare here K. Fischer (p. 85), who applies the term "double meaning" to those witticisms in which both meanings are not equally prominent, but where one overshadows the other. I have applied this term differently. Such a nomenclature is a matter of choice. Usage of speech has rendered no definite decision about them.

We have by this time become familiar with such a large number of different techniques of wit that I am afraid we may lose sight of them. Let us, therefore, attempt to make a summary.

I. CONDENSATION
    (a) with mixed word-formation.
    (b) with modification.

II. THE APPLICATION OF THE SAME MATERIAL
    (c) The whole and the part.
    (d) Change of order.
    (e) Slight modification.
    (f) The same words used in their full or colorless sense.

III. DOUBLE MEANING
    (g) Name and verbal significance.
    (h) Metaphorical and verbal meaning.
    (i) True double meaning (play on words).
    (j) Ambiguous meaning.
    (k) Double meaning with allusion.

This variety causes confusion. It might vex us because we have devoted so much time to the consideration of the technical means of wit, and the stress laid on the forms might possibly arouse our suspicions that we are overvaluing their importance so far as the knowledge of the nature of wit is concerned. But this conjecture is met by the one irrefutable fact: namely, that each time the wit disappears as soon as we remove the effect that was brought to expression by these techniques. We are thus directed to search for the unity in this variety. It must be possible to bring all these techniques under one head. As we have remarked before, it is not difficult to unite the second and third groups, for the double meaning, the play on words, is nothing but the ideal case of utilizing the same material. The latter is here apparently the more comprehensive conception. The examples of dividing, changing the order of the same material, manifold application with slight modifications (c, d, e)—all these could, without difficulty, be subordinated under the conception of double meaning. But what community exists between the technique of the first group— condensation with substitutive formation—and the two other groups—manifold application of the same material?

The Tendency to Economy

It seems to me that this agreement is very simple and clear. The application of the same material is only a special case of condensation and the play on words is nothing but a condensation without substitutive formation. Condensation thus remains as the chief category. A compressing or—to be more exact—an economic tendency controls all these techniques. As Prince Hamlet says: "Thrift, Horatio, thrift." It seems to be all a matter of economy.

Let us examine this economy in individual cases. *"C'est le premier vol de l'aigle."* That is, the first flight of the eagle. Certainly, but it is a depredatious flight. Luckily for the gist of this joke "vol" signifies flight as well as depredation. Has nothing been condensed and economized by this? Certainly, the entire second thought, and it was dropped without any substitution. The double sense of the word "vol" makes such substitution superfluous, or what is just as correct: The word "vol" contains the substitution for the repressed thought without the necessity of supplementing or varying the first sentence. Therein consists the benefit of the double meaning.

Another example: *Gold mine,—gold spoon,* the enormous economy of expression the single word "gold" produces. It really tells the history of two generations in the life of some American families. The father made his fortune through hard toiling in the gold fields during the early pioneer days. The son was born with a golden spoon in his mouth; having been brought up as the son of a wealthy man, he becomes a chronic alcoholic and has to take the gold cure.

Thus there is no doubt that the condensation in these examples produces economy and we shall demonstrate that the same is true in all cases. Where is the economy in such jokes as "*Rousseau—roux et sot*," or "*Antigone— antique-oh-nay*" in which we first failed to find the prime factors in causing us to establish the technique of the manifold application of the same material? In these cases condensation will naturally not cover the ground, but when we exchange it for the broader conception of "economy" we find no difficulty. What we save in such examples as those just given is quite obvious. We save ourselves the trouble of making a criticism, of forming a judgment. Both are contained in the names. The same is true in the "*livelihood*" example and the others thus far analyzed. Where one does not save much is in the example of "*I am in and you are out*," at least the wording of a new answer is saved. The wording of the address, "*I am in*," serves also for the answer. It is little, but in this little lies the wit. The manifold application of the same words in addressing and answering surely comes under the heading of economy. Note how Hamlet sums up the quick succession

of the death of his father and the marriage of
his mother:

> " the funeral baked meats
> Did coldly furnish forth the marriage tables."

But before we accept the " tendency to economize " as the universal character of wit and ask
whence it originates, what it signifies, and how
it gives origin to the resultant pleasure, we shall
concede a doubt which may justly be considered. It may be true that every technique
of wit shows the tendency to economize in expression, but the relationship is not reversible.
Not every economy in expression or every
brevity is witty on that account. We once
raised this question when we still hoped to
demonstrate the condensation process in every
witticism and at that we justly objected by
remarking that a laconism is not necessarily
wit. Hence it must be a peculiar form of
brevity and economy upon which the character
of the wit depends, and just as long as we are
ignorant of this peculiarity the discovery of the
common element in the technique of wit will
bring us no nearer a solution. Besides, we have
the courage to acknowledge that the economies
caused by the technique of wit do not impress us
as very much. They remind one of the manner in which many a housewife economizes

when she spends time and money to reach a distant market because the vegetables can there be had a cent cheaper. What does wit save by means of its technique? Instead of putting together a few new words, which, for the most part, could have been accomplished without any effort, it goes to the trouble of searching for the word which comprises both ideas. Indeed, it must often at first transform the expression of one of the ideas into an unusual form until it furnishes an associative connection with the second thought. Would it not have been simpler, easier, and really more economical to express both thoughts as they happen to come even if no agreement in expression results? Is not the economy in verbal expression more than abrogated through the expenditure of intellectual work? And who economized through it, whom does it benefit? We can temporarily circumvent these doubts by leaving them unsolved until later on. Are we really familiar enough with all the forms of techniques of wit? It will surely be safer to gather new examples and submit them to analysis.

Puns

Indeed, we have not yet given consideration to one of the largest groups into which the techniques of wit may be divided. In this we have perhaps been influenced by the low estimate in which this form of wit is held. It embraces those jokes which are commonly called "puns." These are generally counted as the lowest form of wit, perhaps because they are "cheapest" and can be formed with the least effort. They really make the least demands on the technique of expression just as the actual play on words makes the most. Whereas in the latter both meanings find expression in the identical word, and hence usually in a word used only once, in the pun it is enough if two words for both meanings resemble each other through some slight similarity in structure, in rhythmic consonance, in the community of several vowels, or in some other similar manner. The following examples illustrate these points:

"We are now fallen into that critical age wherein *censores* liberorum are become *censores librorum: Lectores, Lictores.*"

Professor Cromwell says that Rome in exchanging her religion changed *Jupiter* to *Jew Peter.*

It is related that some students wishing to play a trick on Agassiz, the great naturalist, constructed an insect made up of parts taken from different bugs and sent it to him with the question, " What kind of a bug is this?" His answer was " Humbug."

Puns are especially fond of modifying one of the vowels of the word; e.g., Hevesi (*Almanaccando, Reisen in Italien,* p. 87) says of an Italian poet who was hostile to the German emperor, but who was, nevertheless, forced to sing his praises in his hexameters, "*Since he could not exterminate the Cæsars he at least annihilated the cæsuras.*"

From the multitude of puns which are at our disposal it may be of special interest to us to quote a really poor example for which Heine (*Book Le Grand,* Chapter V) is responsible. *After parading for a long time before his lady as an "Indian Prince" the suitor suddenly lays aside his mask and confesses, "Madam, I have lied to you. I have never been in Calcutta any more than that Calcutta roast which I relished yesterday for lunch."* Obviously the fault of this witticism lies in the fact that both words are not merely similar, but identical. The bird which served as a roast for his lunch is called so because it comes from, or at least is supposed to come from, the same city of Calcutta.

K. Fischer has given much attention to this form of wit and insists upon making a sharp distinction between it and the "play on words" (p. 78). "A pun," he says, "is a bad play on words, for it does not play with the word as a word, but merely as a sound." The play on words, however, "transfers itself from the sound of the word into the word itself." On the other hand, he also classifies such jokes as "famillionaire, Antigone (Antique-Oh-nay)," etc., with sound-wit. I see no necessity to follow him in this. In the plays on words, also, the word serves us only as a sound to which this or that meaning attaches itself. Here also usage of language makes no distinction, and when it treats " puns " with disdain but the play on words with a certain respect it seems that these estimations are determined by others as technical viewpoints. One should bear in mind the forms of wit which are referred to as puns. There are persons who have the ability, when they are in a high-spirited mood, to reply with a pun for a long time to every sentence addressed to them. Brill [1] relates that at a gathering some one spoke disparagingly of a certain drama and wound up by saying, "*It was so poor that the first act had to be rewritten.*" "*And now it is rerotten,*" added the punster of the gathering.

At all events we can already infer from the controversies about the line of demarcation between puns and play on words that the former cannot aid us in finding an entirely new tech-

[1] l. c., page 339.

nique of wit. Even if no claims are made for the pun that it utilizes the manifold application of the same material, the accent, nevertheless, falls upon the rediscovering of the familiar and upon the agreement between both words forming the pun. Thus the latter is only a sub-species of the group which reaches its height in the real play on words.

Displacements

There are some witticisms, however, whose techniques baffle almost every attempt to classify them under any of the groups so far investigated. *It is related that while Heine and the poet Soulié were once chatting together in a Parisian drawing-room, there entered one of those Parisians whom one usually compared to Midas, but not alone on account of their money. He was soon surrounded by a crowd which treated him with the greatest deference. " Look over there," said Soulié to Heine, " and see how the nineteenth century is worshipping the Golden Calf." Heine cast one glance upon the object of adoration and replied, as if correcting his friend: " Oh, he must be older than that "* (K. Fischer, p. 82).

Wherein lies the technique of this excellent witticism? According to K. Fischer it lies in the play on words. Thus, for example, he says, "the words 'Golden Calf' may signify Mammon as well as idol-worship,—in the first case the gold is paramount; in the second case it is the animal picture. It may likewise serve to designate in a rather uncomplimentary way one who has very much money and very little brains." If we apply the test and take away the expression "Golden Calf" we naturally also abrogate the wit. We then cause Soulié to say, "Just see how the people are thronging about that blockhead only because he is rich." To be sure, this is no longer witty. Nor would Heine's answer be possible under these circumstances. But let us remember that it is not at all a matter of Soulié's witty comparison, but of Heine's retort, which is surely much more witty. We have then no right to disturb the phrase "the golden calf" which remains as a basis for Heine's words and the reduction can only be applied to the latter. If we dilate upon the words, "Oh, he must be older than that," we can only proceed as follows:

"Oh, he is no longer a calf; he is already a full-grown ox." Heine's wit is therefore based on the fact that he no longer took the "golden calf" metaphorically, but personally by referring it to the moneyed individual himself. If this double meaning is not already contained in the opinion of Soulié!

Let us see. We believe that we can state that this reduction has not altogether destroyed Heine's joke, but, on the contrary, it has left its essential element untouched. It reads as if Soulié were now saying, "Just see how the nineteenth century is worshipping the golden calf," and as if Heine were retorting, "Oh, he is no longer a calf. He is already an ox." And even in this reduced form it is still a witticism. However, another reduction of Heine's words is not possible.

It is a pity that this excellent example contains such complicated technical conditions. And as it cannot aid us toward enlightenment we shall leave it to search for another in which we imagine we can perceive a relationship with the former one.

It is a " bath " joke treating of the dread which some Jews are said to have for bathing. We demand no patent of nobility for our examples nor do we make inquiries about their origin. The only qualifications we require are that they should make us laugh and serve our theoretical interest. It is to be remarked that both these demands are satisfied best by Jewish jokes.

Two Jews meet near a bathing establishment. "Have you taken a bath?" asked one. "How is that?" replies the other. "Is one missing?"

When one laughs very heartily about a joke he is not in the best mood to investigate its technique. It is for this reason that some difficulties are experienced in delving into their analyses. " That is a comic misunderstanding " is the thought that comes to us. Yes, but how about the technique of this joke? Obviously the technique lies in the double meaning of the word *take*. In the first case the word is used in a colorless idiomatic sense, while in the second it is the verb in its full meaning. It is, therefore, a case where the same word is taken now in the " full " and now in the " empty " sense (Group II, f). And if we replace the expression " take a bath " by the simpler equivalent " bathed " the wit disappears. The answer is no longer fitting. The joke, therefore, lies in the expression " take a bath."

This is quite correct, yet it seems that in this case, also, the reduction was applied in the wrong place, for the joke does not lie in the question, but in the answer, or rather in the counter question: " How is that? Is there one missing? " Provided the same is not destroyed the answer cannot be robbed of its wit by any dilation or variation. We also get the impression that in the answer of the second Jew the overlooking of the bath is more significant than the misconception of the word "take." However, here, too, things do not look quite clear and we will, therefore, look for a third example.

Once more we shall resort to a Jewish joke in which, however, the Jewish element is incidental only. Its essence is universally human. It is true that this example, too, contains undesirable complications, but luckily they are not of the kind·so far which have kept us from seeing clearly.

In his distress a needy man borrowed twenty-five dollars from a wealthy acquaintance. The same day he was discovered by his creditor in a restaurant eating a dish of salmon with mayonnaise. The creditor reproached him in these words: " You borrow money from me and then order salmon with mayonnaise. Is that what you needed the money for? " " I don't understand you," responded the debtor, " when I have no money I can't eat salmon with mayonnaise. When I have money I mustn't eat it. Well then, when shall I ever eat salmon with mayonnaise? "

Here we no longer discover any double meaning. Even the repetition of the words " salmon with mayonnaise " cannot contain the technique of the witticism, as it is not the " manifold application of the same material," but an actual, identical repetition required by the context. We may be temporarily nonplussed in this analysis, and, as a pretext, we may wish to dispute the character of the wit in the anecdote which causes us to laugh. What else worthy of notice can be said about the answer of the poor man? It may be supposed that the striking thing about it is its logical character, but, as a matter of fact, the answer is illogical. The debtor endeavors to justify himself for spending the borrowed money on luxuries and asks, with some semblance of right, when he is to be allowed to eat salmon. But this is not at all the correct answer. The creditor does not blame him for eating salmon on the day that he borrowed the money, but reminds him that in his condition he has no right to think of such luxuries at all. The poor *bon vivant* disregards this only possible meaning of the reproach, centers his answer about another point, and acts as if he did not understand the reproach.

Is it possible that the technique of this joke lies in this deviation of the answer from the sense of reproach? A similar changing of the viewpoint—displacement of the psychic accent—may perhaps also be demonstrated in the two previous examples which we felt were related to this one. This can be successfully shown and solves the technique of these examples.

Soulié calls Heine's attention to the fact that
society worships the " golden calf " in the nineteenth century just as the Jewish nation once
did in the desert. To this an answer from
Heine like the following would seem fit: " Yes,
that is human nature. Centuries have changed
nothing in it; " or he might have remarked
something equally apposite. But Heine devi-
ates in his manner from the instigated thought.
Indeed, he does not answer at all. He makes
use of the double meaning found in the phrase
" golden calf " to go off at a tangent. He seizes
upon one of the components of the phrase,
namely, " the calf," and answers as if Soulié's
speech placed the emphasis on it—" Oh, he is
no longer a calf, etc." [1]

The deviation is much more evident in the
bath joke. This example requires a graphic
representation. The first Jew asks, " Have
you taken a *bath?* " The emphasis lies upon
the bath element. The second answers as if the
query were: " Have you *taken* a bath? " The
displacement would have been impossible if
the question had been: " Have you bathed? "
The witless answer would have been: " Bathed?
What do you mean? I don't know what that

---

[1] Heine's answer is a combination of two wit-techniques—a displacement and an allusion—for he does not say directly: " He
is an ox."

means." However, the technique of the wit lies in the displacement of the emphasis from " to bathe " to " to take." [1]

Let us return to the example " salmon with mayonnaise," which is the purest of its kind. What is new in it will direct us into various paths. In the first place we have to give the mechanism of this newly discovered technique. I propose to designate it as having *displacement* for its most essential element. The deviation of the trend of thought consists in displacing the psychic accent to another than the original theme. It is then incumbent upon us to find out the relationship of the technique of displacement to the expression of the witticism. Our example (salmon with mayonnaise) shows us that the displacement technique is absolutely independent of the verbal expression. It does not depend upon words, but upon the mental trend, and to abrogate it we are not helped by substitution so long as the sense of the answer is adhered to. The reduction is possible only when we change the

---

[1] The word "take," owing to its meanings, lends itself very well towards the formation of plays upon words, a pure example of which I wish to cite as a contrast to the displacement mentioned above. While walking with his friend, in front of a café, a well-known stock-plunger and bank director made this proposal: "Let us go in and take something." His friend held him back and said: "My dear sir, remember there are people in there."

mental trend and permit the gastronomist to answer directly to the reproach which he eluded in the conception of the joke. The reduced conception will then be: " What I like I cannot deny myself, and it is all the same to me where I get the money for it. Here you have my explanation as to why I happen to be eating salmon with mayonnaise today just after you have loaned me some money." But that would not be a witticism but a *cynicism*. It will be instructive to compare this joke with one which is closely allied to it in meaning.

A man who was addicted to drink supported himself in a small city by giving lessons. His vice gradually became known and he lost most of his pupils in consequence. A friend of his took it upon himself to admonish him to reform. " Look here," he said, " you could have the best scholars in town if you would give up drinking. Why not do it? " " What are you talking about? " was the indignant reply. " I am giving lessons in order to be able to drink. Shall I give up drinking in order to obtain scholars? "

This joke, too, carries the stamp of logic which we have noted in the case of " salmon with mayonnaise," but it is no longer displacement-wit. The answer is a direct one. The cynicism, which is veiled there, is openly admitted here, " For me drink is the most important thing." The technique of this witticism is really very poor and cannot explain its effect. It lies merely in the change in order of the same material, or to be more exact, in the reversal of the means-and-end relationship between drink and giving lessons or getting scholars. As I gave no greater emphasis in the reduction to this factor of the expression the witticism is somewhat blurred; it may be expressed as follows: " What a senseless demand to make. For me, drink is the most important thing and not the scholars. Giving lessons is only a means towards more drink." The wit is really dependent upon the expression.

In the bath wit, the dependence of the witticism upon the wording " have you taken a bath " is unmistakable and a change in the wording nullifies the joke. The technique in this case is quite complicated. It is a combination of double meaning (sub-group f) and displacement. The wording of the question admits a double meaning. The joke arises from the fact that the answer is given not in the sense expected by the questioner, but has a different subordinate sense. By making the displacement retrogressive we are accordingly in position to find a reduction which leaves the double meaning in the expression and still does away with the wit.

"*Have you taken a bath?*" "*Taken what? A bath? What is that?*" But that is no longer a witticism, It is simply either a spiteful or playful exaggeration.

In Heine's joke about the " golden calf " the double meaning plays a quite similar part. It makes it possible for the answer to deviate from the instigated stream of thought—a thing which happens in the joke about " salmon and mayonnaise "—without any such dependence upon the wording. In the reduction Soulié's speech and Heine's answer would be as follows: " It reminds one very much of the worship of the golden calf when one sees the people throng around that man simply because he is rich." Heine's answer would be: " That he is made so much of on account of his wealth is not the worst part. You do not emphasize enough the fact that his ignorance is forgiven on account of his wealth." Thus, while the double meaning would be retained the displacement-wit would be eliminated.

Here we may be prepared for the objection which might be raised, namely, that we are seeking to tear asunder these delicate differentiations which really belong together. Does not every double meaning furnish occasion for

displacement and for a deviation of the stream
of thought from one sense to another? And
shall we agree that a "double meaning" and
"displacement" should be designated as rep-
resentatives of two entirely different types of
wit? It is true that a relation between double
meaning and displacement actually exists, but
it has nothing to do with our differentiation
of the techniques of wit. In cases of double
meaning the wit contains nothing but a word
capable of several interpretations which allows
the hearer to find the transition from one
thought to another, and which with a little
forcing may be compared to a displacement.
In the cases of displacement-wit, however, the
witticism itself contains a stream of thought
in which the displacement is brought about.
Here the displacement belongs to the work
which is necessary for its understanding.
Should this differentiation not be clear to us we
can make use of the reduction method, which is
an unfailing way for tangible demonstration.
We do not deny, however, that there is something in this objection. It calls our attention
to the fact that we cannot confuse the psychic
processes in the formation of wit (the wit-work)
with the psychic processes in the conception of
the wit (the understanding-work). The object

of our present investigation will be confined only to the former.[1]

Are there still other examples of the technique of displacement? They are not easily found, but the following witticism is a very good specimen. It also shows a lack of over-emphasized logic found in our former examples.

A horse-dealer in recommending a saddle horse to his client said: " If you mount this horse at four o'clock in the morning you will be in Monticello at six-thirty in the morning." " What will I do in Monticello at six-thirty in the morning? " asked the client.

Here the displacement is very striking. The horse-dealer mentions the early arrival in the small city only with the obvious intention of proving the efficiency of the horse. The client disregards the capacity of the animal, about which he evidently has no more doubts, and takes up only the data of the example selected

---

[1] For the latter see a later chapter. It will perhaps not be superfluous to add here a few words for better understanding. The displacement regularly occurs between a statement and an answer, and turns the stream of thought to a direction different from the one started in the statement. The justification for separating the displacement from the double meaning is best seen in the examples where both are combined, that is, where the wording of the statement admits of a double meaning which was not intended by the speaker, but which reveals in the answer the way to the displacement (see examples).

for the test. The reduction of this joke is comparatively simple.

More difficulties are encountered by another
example, the technique of which is very obscure.
It can be solved, however, through the application of double meaning with displacement. The
joke relates the subterfuge employed by a
" schadchen " (Jewish marriage broker). It
belongs to a class which will claim more of our
attention later.

*The " schadchen " had assured the suitor
that the father of the girl was no longer living.
After the engagement had been announced the
news leaked out that the father was still living
and serving a sentence in prison. The suitor
reproached the agent for deceiving him.
" Well," said the latter, " what did I tell you?
Do you call that living? "*

The double meaning lies in the word " living,"
and the displacement consists in the fact that
the " schadchen " avoids the common meaning
of the word, which is a contrast to " death," and
uses it in the colloquial sense: " You don't call
that living." In doing this he explains his
former utterance as a double meaning, although
this manifold application is here quite out of
place. Thus far the technique resembles that
of the " golden calf " and the " bath " jokes.
Here, however, another factor comes into con-

sideration which disturbs the understanding of the technique through its obtrusiveness. One might say that this joke is a "characterization-wit." It endeavors to illustrate by example the marriage agent's characteristic admixture of mendacious impudence and repartee. We shall learn that this is only the "show-side" of the façade of the witticism, that is, its sense. Its object serves a different purpose. We shall also defer our attempt at reduction.[1]

After these complicated examples, which are not at all easy to analyze, it will be gratifying to find a perfectly pure and transparent example of "displacement-wit." *A beggar implored the help of a wealthy baron for a trip to Ostend, where he asserted the physicians had ordered him to take sea baths for his health. "Very well, I shall assist you," said the rich baron, " but is it absolutely necessary for you to go to Ostend, which is the most expensive of all watering-places?" "Sir," was the reproving reply, " nothing is too expensive for my health."* Certainly that is a proper attitude, but hardly proper for the supplicant. The answer is given from the viewpoint of a rich man. The beggar acts as if it were his own money that he was willing to sacrifice for his health, as if money and health concerned the *same* person.

[1] See Chapter III.

Nonsense as a Technical Means

Let us take up again in this connection the instructive example of "salmon with mayonnaise." It also presents to us a side in which we noticed a striking display of logical work and we have learned from analyzing it that this logic concealed an error of thought, namely, a displacement of the stream of thought. Henceforth, even if only by way of contrast association, we shall be reminded of other jokes which, on the contrary, present clearly something contradictory, something nonsensical, or foolish. We shall be curious to discover wherein the technique of the witticism lies. I shall first present the strongest and at the same time the purest example of the entire group. Once more it is a Jewish joke.

Ike was serving in the artillery corps. He was seemingly an intelligent lad, but he was unwieldy and had no interest in the service. One of his superiors, who was kindly disposed toward him, drew him aside and said to him: "Ike, you are out of place among us. I would advise you to buy a cannon and make yourself independent."

The advice, which makes us laugh heartily, is obvious nonsense. There are no cannon to be bought and an individual cannot possibly

make himself independent as a fighting force
or establish himself, as it were. One cannot
remain one minute in doubt but that this advice is not pure nonsense, but witty nonsense
and an excellent joke. By what means does
the nonsense become a witticism?

We need not meditate very long. From the
discussions of the authors in the Introduction
we can guess that sense lurks in such witty
nonsense, and that this sense in nonsense trans-
forms nonsense into wit. In our example the
sense is easily found. The officer who gives
the artilleryman, Ike, the nonsensical advice
pretends to be stupid in order to show Ike how
stupidly he is acting. He imitates Ike as if to
say, " I will now give you some advice which is
exactly as stupid as you are." He enters into
Ike's stupidity and makes him conscious of it by
making it the basis of a proposition which must
meet with Ike's wishes, for if Ike owned a cannon and took up the art of warfare on his own
account, of what advantage would his intelligence and ambition be to him? How would
he take care of the cannon and acquaint
himself with its mechanism in order to meet
the competition of other possessors of cannon?

I am breaking off the analysis of this example
to show the same sense in nonsense in a shorter

and simpler, though less glaring case of non-sense-wit.

"*Never to be born would be best for mortal man.*" "*But,*" added the sages of the *Fliegende Blätter,* "*hardly one man in a hundred thousand has this luck.*"

The modern appendix to the ancient philosophical saying is pure nonsense, and becomes still more stupid through the addition of the seemingly careful "hardly." But this appendix in attaching itself to the first sentence incontestably and correctly limits it. It can thus open our eyes to the fact that that piece of wisdom so reverently scanned, is neither more nor less than sheer nonsense. He who is not born of woman is not mortal; for him there exists no " good " and no " best." The nonsense of the joke, therefore, serves here to expose and present another bit of nonsense as in the case of the artilleryman. Here I can add a third example which, owing to its context, scarcely deserves a detailed description. It serves, however, to illustrate the use of non-sense in wit in order to represent another element of nonsense.

A man about to go upon a journey intrusted his daughter to his friend, begging him to watch over her chastity during his absence. When he returned some months later he found that she was pregnant. Naturally he reproached his friend. The latter alleged that he could not explain this unfortunate occurrence. " Where has she been sleeping? " the father finally asked. " In the same room with my son," replied the friend. " How is it that you allowed her to sleep in the same room with your son after I had begged you so earnestly to take good care of her? " remonstrated the father. " Well," explained the friend, " there was a screen between them. There was your daughter's bed and over there was my son's bed and between them stood the screen." " And suppose he went behind the screen? What then? " asked the parent. " Well, in that case," rejoined the friend thoughtfully, " it might be possible."

In this joke—aside from the other qualities of this poor witticism—we can easily get the reduction. Obviously, it would read like this: " You have no right to reproach me. How could you be so foolish as to leave your daughter in a house where she must live in the constant companionship of a young man? As if it were possible for a stranger to be responsible for the chastity of a maiden under such circumstances! " The seeming stupidity of the friend here also serves as a reflection of the stupidity of the father. By means of the reduction we have eliminated the nonsense contained in the witticism as well as the witticism itself. We have not gotten rid of the " nonsense " element itself, as it finds another place in the context of the sentence after it has been reduced to its true meaning.

We can now also attempt the reduction of the joke about the cannon. The officer might have said: " I know, Ike. that you are an intelligent business man, but I must tell you that you are very stupid if you do not realize that one cannot act in the army as one does in business, where each one is out for himself and competes with the other. Military service demands subordination and co-operation."

The technique of the nonsense witticisms hitherto discussed really consists in advancing something apparently absurd or nonsensical which, however, discloses a sense serving to illustrate and represent some other actual absurdity and nonsense.

Has the employment of contradiction in the technique of wit always this meaning? Here is another example which answers this affirmatively. On an occasion when Phocion's speech was applauded he turned to his friends and asked: *" Did I say something foolish? "*

This question seems paradoxical, but we immediately comprehend its meaning. " What have I said that has pleased this stupid crowd?

I ought really to be ashamed of the applause, for if it appealed to these fools, it could not have been very clever after all."

Other examples teach us that absurdity is used very often in the technique of wit without serving at all the purpose of uncovering another piece of nonsense.

A well-known university teacher who was wont to spice richly with jokes his rather dry specialty was once congratulated upon the birth of his youngest son, who was bestowed upon him at a rather advanced age. "Yes," said he to the well-wishers, " it is remarkable what mortal hands can accomplish." This reply seems especially meaningless and out of place, for children are called the blessings of God to distinguish them from creations of mortal hands. But it soon dawns upon us that this answer has a meaning and an obscene one at that. The point in question is not that the happy father wishes to appear stupid in order to make something else or some other persons appear stupid. The seemingly senseless answer causes us astonishment. It puzzles us, as the authors would have it. We have seen that the authors deduce the entire mechanism of such jokes from the change of the succession of " clearness and confusion." We shall try to form an opinion about this later. Here we content ourselves by remarking that the technique of this witticism consists in advancing such confusing and senseless elements.

An especially peculiar place among the nonsense jokes is assumed by this joke of Lichtenberg.

"*He was surprised that the two holes were cut in the pelts of cats just where their eyes were located.*" It is certainly foolish to be surprised about something that is obvious in itself, something which is really the explanation of an identity. It reminds one of a seriously intended utterance of Michelet (*The Woman*) which, as I remember it, runs as follows: "*How beautifully everything is arranged by nature. As soon as the child comes into the world it finds a mother who is ready to care for it.*" This utterance of Michelet is really silly, but the one of Lichtenberg is a witticism, which makes use of the absurdity for some purpose. There is something behind it. What? At present that is something we cannot discuss.

Sophistic Faulty Thinking

We have learned from two groups of examples that the wit-work makes use of deviations from normal thought, namely, *displacement* and *absurdity*, as technical means of pre-

senting witty expressions. It is only just to
expect that other faulty thinking may find a
similar application. Indeed, a few examples of
this sort can be cited.

*A gentleman entered a shop and ordered a
fancy cake, which, however, he soon returned,
asking for some liqueur in its stead. He drank
the liqueur, and was about to leave without
paying for it. The shopkeeper held him back.
"What do you want of me?" he asked.
"Please pay for the liqueur," said the shopkeeper. "But I have given you the fancy cake
for it." "Yes, but you have not paid for that
either." "Well, neither have I eaten it."*

This little story also bears the semblance of
logic which we already know as the suitable
façade for faulty thinking. The error, obviously, lies in the fact that the cunning customer establishes a connection between the return of the fancy cake and its exchange for the
liqueur, a connection which really does not
exist. The state of affairs may be divided into
two processes which as far as the shopkeeper
is concerned are independent of each other.
He first took the fancy cake and returned it,
so that he owes nothing for it. He then took
the liqueur, for which he owes money. One
might say that the customer uses the relation
"for it" in a double sense, or, to speak more

correctly, by means of a double sense he forms a relation which does not hold in reality.[1]

The opportunity now presents itself for making a not unimportant confession. We are here busying ourselves with an investigation of technique of wit by means of examples, and we ought to be sure that the examples which we have selected are really true witticisms. The facts are, however, that in a series of cases we fall into doubt as to whether or not the example in question may be called a joke. We have no criterion at our disposal before investigation itself furnishes one. Usage of language is unreliable and is itself in need of examination for its authority. To decide the question we can rely on nothing else but a certain " feeling," which we may interpret by saying that in our judgment the decision follows certain criteria which are not yet accessible to our knowledge. We shall naturally not appeal to this " feeling " for substantial proof. In the case of the last-mentioned example we cannot help doubting whether we may present it as a witticism, as a sophistical witticism, or

---

[1] A similar nonsense technique results when the joke aims to maintain a connection which seems to be removed through the special conditions of its content. A joke of this sort is related by J. Falke (1. c.): " *Is this the place where the Duke of Wellington spoke these words?* " " *Yes, this is the place; but he never spoke these words.* "

merely as a sophism. The fact is that we do not yet know wherein the character of wit lies.

On the other hand the following example, which evinces, as it were, the complementary faulty thinking, is a witticism without any doubt. Again it is a story of a marriage agent. *The agent is defending the girl he has proposed against the attacks of her prospective fiancé. "The mother-in-law does not suit me," the latter remarks. "She is a crabbed, foolish person." "That's true," replies the agent, "but you are not going to marry the mother-in-law, but the daughter." "Yes, but she is no longer young, and she is not pretty, either." "That's nothing: if she is not young or pretty you can trust her all the more." "But she hasn't much money." "Why talk of money? Are you going to marry money? You want a wife, don't you?" "But she is a hunchback." "Well, what of that? Do you expect her to have no blemishes at all?"*

It is really a question of an ugly girl who is no longer young, who has a paltry dowry and a repulsive mother, and who is besides equipped with a pretty bad deformity, relations which are not at all inviting to matrimony. The marriage agent knows how to present each individual fault in a manner to cause one to become reconciled to it, and then takes up the unpardonable hunch back as the one fault which can be excused in any one. Here again there is the semblance of logic which is characteristic of sophisms, and which serves to conceal the faulty thinking. It is apparent that the girl possesses nothing but faults, many of which can be overlooked, but one that cannot be passed by. The chances for the marriage become very slim. The agent acts as if he removed each individual fault by his evasions, forgetting that each leaves behind some depreciation which is added to the next one. He insists upon dealing with each factor individually, and refuses to combine them into a sum-total.

A similar omission forms the nucleus of another sophism which causes much laughter, though one can well question its right to be called a joke.

A. had borrowed a copper kettle from B., and upon returning it was sued by B. because it had a large hole which rendered it unserviceable. His defense was this: " In the first place I never borrowed any kettle from B., secondly the kettle had a hole in it when I received it from B., thirdly the kettle was in perfect condition when I returned it." Each separate protest is good by itself, but taken together they exclude each other. A. treats individually what must be taken as a whole, just as the marriage agent when he deals with the imperfections of the bride.   One can also say that A. uses " and " where only an " either—or " is possible.

Another sophism greets us in the following marriage agent story. *The suitor objects because the bride has a short leg and therefore limps. The agent contradicts him. " You are wrong," he says. " Suppose you marry a woman whose legs are sound and straight. What do you gain by it? You are not sure from day to day that she will not fall down, break a leg, and then be lame for the rest of her life. Just consider the pain, the excitement, and the doctor's bill. But if you marry this one nothing can happen. Here you have a finished job."*

Here the semblance of logic is very shallow, for no one will by any means admit that a " finished misfortune " is to be preferred to a mere possibility of such.   The error in the stream of thought will be seen more easily in a second example.

In the temple of Cracow sat the great Rabbi N. praying with his disciples. Suddenly he emitted a cry and in response to his troubled disciples said: " The great Rabbi L. died just now in Lemberg." The congregation thereupon went into mourning for the deceased. In the

course of the next day travelers from Lemberg
were asked how the rabbi had died, and what
had caused his death. They knew nothing
about the event, however, as, they said, they
had left him in the best of health. Finally it
was definitely ascertained that the Rabbi of
Lemberg had not died at the hour on which
Rabbi N. had felt his death telepathically, and
that he was still living. A stranger seized the
opportunity to banter a pupil of the Cracow
rabbi about the episode. "That was a glorious
exhibition that your rabbi made of himself
when he saw the Rabbi of Lemberg die," he
said. "Why, the man is still living!" "No
matter," replied the pupil. "To look from
Cracow to Lemberg was wonderful anyhow."

Here the faulty thinking common to both
of the last examples is openly shown. The
value of fanciful ideas is unfairly matched
against reality; possibility is made equivalent
to actuality. To look from Cracow to Lemberg despite the miles between would have been
an imposing telepathic feat had it resulted in
some truth, but the disciple gives no heed to
that. It might have been possible that the
Rabbi of Lemberg had died at the moment
when the Rabbi of Cracow had proclaimed his
death, but the pupil displaces the accent from
the condition under which the teacher's act

would be remarkable to the unconditional admiration of this act. " *In magnis rebus voluisse sat est* " is a similar point of view. Just as in this example reality is sacrificed in favor of possibility, so in the foregoing example the marriage agent suggests to the suitor that the possibility of the woman's becoming lame through an accident is a far more important consideration to be taken into account; whereas the question as to whether or not she is lame is put altogether into the background.

Automatic Errors of Thought

Another interesting group attaches itself to this one of sophistical faulty thinking, a group in which the faulty thinking may be designated as *automatic*. It is perhaps only a stroke of fate that all of the examples which I shall cite for this new group are again stories referring to marriage agents.

The agent brought along an assistant to a conference about a bride. This assistant was to confirm his assertions. " She is as well made as a pine tree," said the agent. " Like a pine tree," repeated the echo. " She has eyes which one must appreciate." " Wonderful eyes," confirmed the echo. " She is cultured beyond words. She possesses extraordinary culture."

" Wonderfully cultured," repeated the assistant.
" However, one thing is true," confessed the
agent. " She has a slight hunch on her back."
" And what a hunch!" confirmed the echo.

The other stories are quite analogous to this
one, but they are cleverer.

On being introduced to his prospective bride
the suitor was rather unpleasantly surprised,
and drawing aside the marriage agent he re-
proachfully whispered to him: " Why have you
brought me here? She is ugly and old. She
squints, has bad teeth, and bleary eyes."
" You can talk louder," interrupted the agent.
" She is deaf, too."

A prospective bridegroom made his first call
on his future bride in company with the agent,
and while in the parlor waiting for the appear-
ance of the family the agent drew the young
man's attention to a glass closet containing a
handsome silver set. " Just look at these
things," he said. " You can see how wealthy
these people are." " But is it not possible that
these articles were just borrowed for the occa-
sion," inquired the suspicious young man, " so
as to give the appearance of wealth?" " What
an idea," answered the agent protestingly.
" Who in the world would lend them any-
thing?"

In all three cases one finds the same thing.

A person who reacts several times in succession in the same manner continues in the same manner on the next occasion where it becomes unsuited and runs contrary to his intentions. Falling into the automatism of habit he fails to adapt himself to the demands of the situation. Thus in the first story the assistant forgot that he was taken along in order to influence the suitor in favor of the proposed bride, and as he had thus far accomplished his task by emphasizing through repetition the excellencies attributed to the lady, he now emphasizes also her timidly conceded hunch back which he should have belittled.

The marriage agent in the second story is so fascinated by the failings and infirmities of the bride that he completes the list from his own knowledge, which it was certainly neither his business nor his intention to do. Finally in the third story he is so carried away by his zeal to convince the young man of the family's wealth that in order to corroborate his proofs he blurts out something which must upset all his efforts. Everywhere the automatism triumphs over the appropriate variation of thought and expression.

That is quite easy to understand, although it must cause confusion when it is brought to our attention that these three stories could just

as well be termed "comical" as "witty." Like
every act of unmasking and self-betrayal the
discovery of the psychic automatism also belongs to technique of the comic. We suddenly
see ourselves here confronted with the problem
of the relationship of wit to the comic element—
a subject which we endeavored to avoid (see
the Introduction). Are these stories only
"comical" and not "witty" also? Does the
comic element employ here the same means as
does the wit? And again, of what does the
peculiar character of wit consist?

We must adhere to the fact that the technique of the group of witticisms examined last
consists of nothing else but the establishment of
"faulty thinking." We are forced to admit,
however, that so far the investigation has led
us further into darkness than to illumination.
Nevertheless we do not abandon the hope of
arriving at a result by means of a more thorough knowledge of the technique of wit which
may become the starting-point for further insight.

Unification

The next examples of wit with which we wish
to continue our investigation do not give us as
much work. Their technique reminds us very
much of what we already know. Here is one

of Lichtenberg's jokes. *"January,"* he says, *" is the month in which one extends good wishes to his friends, and the rest are months in which the good wishes are not fulfilled."*

As these witticisms may be called clever rather than strong, we shall reinforce the impression by examining a few more.

" Human life is divided into two halves; during the first one looks forward to the second, and during the second one looks backward to the first."

" Experience consists in experiencing what one does not care to experience." (The last two examples were cited by K. Fischer.)

One cannot help being reminded by these examples of a group, treated of before, which is characterized by the " manifold application of the same material." The last example especially will cause us to ask why we have not inserted it there instead of presenting it here in a new connection. " Experience " is described through its own terms just as some of the examples cited above. Neither would I be against this correction. However, I am of the opinion that the other two cases, which are surely similar in character, contain a different factor which is more striking and more important than the manifold application of the same word which shows nothing here touching upon double meaning. And what is more, I wish to emphasize that new and unexpected identities are here formed which show themselves in relations of ideas to one another, in relations of definitions to each other, or to a common third. I would call this process *unification*. Obviously it is analogous to condensation by compression into similar words. Thus the two halves of human life are described by the inter-relationship discovered between them: during the first part one longs for the second, and in the second one longs for the first. To speak more precisely there were two relationships very similar to each other which were selected for description. The similarity of the relationship that corresponds to the similarity of the words which, just for this reason, might recall the manifold application of the same material—(looks forward)

(looks backward).

In Lichtenberg's joke, January and the months contrasted with it are characterized again by a modified relationship to a third factor: these are good wishes which one receives in the first month, but are not fulfilled during the other months. The differentiation from the manifold application of the same material which is really related to double meaning is here quite clear.

A good example of unification-wit needing no explanation is the following:

J. B. Rousseau, the French poet, wrote an ode to posterity (à la postérité). *Voltaire, thinking that the poor quality of the poem in no way justified its reaching posterity, wittily remarked, "This poem will not reach its destination"* (K. Fischer).

The last example may remind us of the fact that it is essentially unification which forms the basis of the so-called repartee in wit. For ready repartee consists in using the defense for aggression and in "turning the tables" or in "paying with the same coin." That is, the repartee consists in establishing an unexpected identity between attack and counter-attack.

For example, *a baker said to a tavern keeper, one of whose fingers was festering: "I guess your finger got into your beer." The tavern keeper replied: "You are wrong. One of your rolls got under my finger nail"* (Ueberhorst: *Das Komische*, II, 1900).

While Serenissimus was traveling through his domains he noticed a man in the crowds who bore a striking resemblance to himself. He beckoned him to come over and asked: *"Was your mother ever employed in my home?" "No, sire,"* replied the man, *"but my father was."*

While Duke Karl of Würtemberg was riding horseback he met a dyer working at his trade. *" Can you color my white horse blue? " " Yes, sire,"* was the rejoinder, *" if the animal can stand the boiling! "*

In this excellent repartee, which answers a foolish question with a condition that is equally impossible, there occurs another technical factor which would have been omitted if the dyer's reply had been: " No, sire, I am afraid that the horse could not stand being boiled."

Another peculiarly interesting technical means at the disposal of unification is the addition of the conjunction " and." Such correlation signifies a connection which could not be understood otherwise. When Heine (*Harzreise*) says of the city of Göttingen, *" In general the inhabitants of Göttingen are divided into students, professors, Philistines, and cattle,"* we understand this combination exactly in the sense which he furthermore emphasized by adding: " These four social groups are distinguished little less than sharply." Again, when he speaks about the school where he had to submit *" to so much Latin, drubbing, and geography,"* he wants to convey by this combination, which is made very conspicuous by placing the drubbing between the two studies, that the schoolboy's conception unmistakably described by the drub-

THE TECHNIQUE OF WIT

bing should be extended also to Latin and geography.

In Lipps's book we find among the examples of "witty enumeration" (Koordination) the following verse, which stands nearest to Heine's "students, professors, Philistines, and cattle."

" With a fork and with much effort his mother pulled him from a mess."

" As if effort were an instrument like the fork," adds Lipps by way of explanation. But we get the impression that there is nothing witty in this sentence. To be sure it is very comical, whereas Heine's co-ordination is un- doubtedly witty. We shall, perhaps, recall these examples later when we shall no longer be forced to evade the problem of the relationship between wit and the comic.

Representation Through the Opposite

We have remarked in the example of the Duke and the dyer that it would still have been a joke by means of unification had the dyer replied, " No, I fear that the horse could not stand being boiled." In substituting a " yes " for the " no " which rightly belonged there, we meet a new technical means of wit the applica- tion of which we shall study in other examples.

This joke, which resembles the one we have

just cited from K. Fischer, is somewhat simpler. *"Frederick the Great heard of a Silesian clergyman who had the reputation of communicating with spirits. He sent for him and received him with the following question: 'Can you call up ghosts?' 'At your pleasure, your majesty,' replied the clergyman, 'but they won't come.'"* Here it is perfectly obvious that the wit lies in the substitution of its opposite for the only possible answer, " No." To complete this substitution " but " had to be added to " yes," so that " yes " plus " but " gives the equivalent for " no."

This " representation through the opposite," as we choose to call it, serves the mechanism of wit in several ways. In the following cases it appears almost in its pure form:

" This woman resembles Venus de Milo in many points. Like her she is extraordinarily old, has no teeth, and has white spots on the yellow surface of her body " (Heine).

Here ugliness is depicted by making it agree with the most beautiful. Of course these agreements consist of attributes expressed in double meaning or of matters of slight importance. The latter applies to the second example.

" The attributes of the greatest men were all united in himself. Like Alexander his head was tilted to one side: like Cæsar he always had

something in his hair. He could drink coffee like Leibnitz, and once settled in his armchair he forgot eating and drinking like Newton, and like him had to be awakened. He wore a wig like Dr. Johnson, and like Cervantes the fly of his trousers was always open " (Lichtenberg: *The Great Mind*).

J. V. Falke's *Lebenserinnerungen an eine Reise nach Ireland* (page 271) furnishes an exceptionally good example of "representation through the opposite" in which the use of words of a double meaning plays absolutely no part. The scene is laid in a wax figure museum, like Mme. Tussaud's. A lecturer discourses on one figure after another to his audience, which is composed of old and young people. " *This is the Duke of Wellington and his horse,*" he says. Whereupon a young girl remarks, " *Which is the duke and which is the horse?* " " *Just as you like, my pretty child,*" is the reply. " *You pay your money and you take your choice.*"

The reduction of this Irish joke would be: " It is gross impudence on the part of the museum's management to offer such an exhibition to the public. It is impossible to distinguish between the horse and the rider (playful exaggeration), and it is for this exhibit that one pays one's hard-earned money! " The indignant expression is now dramatized and applied to a trivial occurrence. In the place of the entire audience there appears one woman and the riding figure becomes individually determined. It is necessarily the Duke of Wellington, who is so very popular in Ireland. But the insolence of the museum proprietor or lecturer who takes money from the public and offers nothing in return is represented by the opposite, through a speech, in which he extols himself as a conscientious business man whose fondest desire is to respect the rights to which the public is entitled through the admission fee. One then realizes that the technique of this joke is not very simple. In so far as a way is found to allow the swindler to assert his scrupulosity it may be said that the joke is a case of "representation through the opposite." The fact, however, that he does it on an occasion where something different is demanded of him, and the fact that he replies in terms of commercial integrity when he is expected to discuss the similarity of the figures, shows that it is a case of displacement. The technique of the joke lies in the combination of both technical means.

Outdoing-wit

This example is closely allied to another small group which might be called "outdoing-wit." Here "yes," which would be proper in the reduction, is replaced by "no," which, owing to its context, is equivalent to a still stronger "yes." The same mechanism holds true when the case is reversed. The contradiction takes the place of an exaggerated confirmation. An example of this nature is seen in the following epigram from Lessing.[1]

" The good Galathee! 'Tis said that she dyes her hair black, yet it was black when she bought it."

Lichtenberg's make-believe mocking defense of philosophy is another example.

" There are more things in heaven and earth than are dreamt of in your philosophy," Prince Hamlet had disdainfully declared. Lichtenberg well knew that this condemnation was by no means severe enough, in that it does not take into account all that can be said against philosophy. He therefore added the following: *" But there is also much in philosophy which is found neither in heaven nor on earth."* To be sure, his assertion supplements what was lacking in Hamlet's philosophical utterance, but in doing this he adds another and still greater reproach.

More transparent still, because they show no trace of displacement, are two Jewish

---

[1] Following an example of the *Greek Anthology.*

jokes which are, however, of the coarse kind.

Two Jews were conversing about bathing. " I take a bath once a year," said one, " whether I need one or not."

It is clear that this boastful assurance of his cleanliness only betrays his state of uncleanliness.

A Jew noticed remnants of food on the beard of another. " I can tell you what you ate yesterday," he remarked. " Well, let's hear it," said another. " Beans," said the first one. " You are wrong," responded the other. " I had beans the day before yesterday."

The following example is an excellent " outdoing " witticism which can be traced easily to representation through the opposite.

The king condescended to pay a visit at a surgical clinic, and found the professor of surgery engaged in amputating a leg. He watched the various steps of the operation with interest and expressed his royal approval with these loud utterances: " Bravo, bravo, Professor." When the operation was over the professor approached the king, bowed low, and asked: " Does your majesty also command the amputation of the other leg?"

Whatever the professor may have thought during this royal applause surely could not have been expressed unchanged. His real thoughts were: "Judging by this applause he must be under the impression that I am amputating the poor devil's diseased leg by order of and for the pleasure of the king. To be sure, I have other reasons for performing this operation." But instead of expressing these thoughts he goes to the king and says: "I have no other reasons but your majesty's order for performing this operation. The applause you accorded me has inspired me so much that I am only awaiting your majesty's command to amputate the other leg also." He thus succeeded in making himself understood by expressing the opposite of what he really thought but had to keep to himself. Such an expression of the opposite represents an incredible exaggeration or outdoing.

As we gather from these examples, representation through the opposite is a means frequently and effectively used in the technique of wit. We need not overlook, however, something else, namely, that this technique is by no means confined only to wit. When Marc Antony, after his long speech in the Forum had changed the mood of the mob listening to Cæsar's obsequies, at last repeats the words,

"For Brutus was an honorable man,"

he well knows that the mob will scream the true meaning of his words at him, namely,

"They are traitors: nice honorable men!"

Or when *Simplicissimus* transcribes a collection of unheard-of brutalities and cynicisms as expressions of "people with temperaments," this, too, is a representation through the opposite. However, this is no longer designated as wit, but as "irony." Indeed, the only technique that is characteristic of irony is representation through the opposite. Besides, one reads and hears about "ironical wit." Hence there is no longer any doubt that technique alone is not capable of characterizing wit. There must be something else which we have not yet discovered. On the other hand, however, the fact that the reduction of the technique destroys the wit still remains uncontradicted. For the present it may be difficult for us to unite for the explanation of wit the two strong points which we have already gained.

Indirect Expression

Since representation through the opposite belongs to the technical means of wit, we may also expect that wit could make use of its reverse, namely, the representation through the similar and cognate. Indeed, when we continue our investigation we find that this forms the technique of a new and especially extensive group of thought-witticisms. We can describe the peculiarity of this technique much better if instead of representation through the " cognate " we use the expression representation through " relationships and associations." We shall start with the last characteristic and illustrate it by an example.

Indirect Expression with Allusion

It is an American anecdote and runs as follows. *By undertaking a series of risky schemes, two not very scrupulous business men had succeeded in amassing an enormous fortune and were now intent on forcing their way into good society. Among other things they thought it advisable to have their portraits painted by the most prominent and most expensive painters in the city, men whose works were considered masterpieces. The costly pictures were exhibited for the first time at a great evening gathering, and the hosts themselves led the most prominent connoisseur and art critic to the wall of the salon on which both portraits were hanging side by side, in order to elicit from him a favorable criticism. He examined the portraits for a long time, then shook his*

*head as if he were missing something. At
length he pointed to the bare space between
the pictures, and asked, "And where is the
Savior?"*

The meaning of this expression is clear. It
is again the expression of something which cannot be represented directly. In what way does
this "indirect expression" come about? By a
series of very obvious associations and conclusions let us work backwards from the verbal
setting.

The query, *"where is the Savior?"* or *"where
is the picture of the Savior?"* arouses the conjecture that the two pictures have reminded the
speaker of a similar arrangement familiar to
him as it is familiar to us. This arrangement,
of which one element is here missing, shows the
figure of the Savior between two other figures.
There is only one such case: Christ hanging
between the two thieves. The missing element
is emphasized by the witticism, and the similarity rests in the figures at the right and left of
the Savior, which are not mentioned in the jest.
It can only mean that the pictures hanging in
the drawing-room are likewise those of thieves.
This is what the critic wished to, but could
not say, "You are a pair of scoundrels," or
more in detail, "What do I care about your
portraits? You are a pair of scoundrels, that

I know." And by means of a few associations and conclusive inferences he has said it in a manner which we designate as "allusion."

We immediately remember that we have encountered the process of allusion before. Namely, in double meaning, when one of the two meanings expressed by the same word stands out very prominently because being used much oftener and more commonly, our attention is directed to it first, whereas the other meaning remains in the background because it is more remote—such cases we wished to describe as double meaning with allusion. In an entire series of examples which we have hitherto examined, we have remarked that their technique is not simple and we realized that the process of allusion was the factor that complicated it. For example, see the contradiction-witticism in which the congratulations on the birth of the youngest child are acknowledged by the remark that it is remarkable what human hands can accomplish (p. 77).

In the American anecdote we have the process of allusion without the double meaning, and we find that the character of this process consists in completing the picture through mental association. It is not difficult to guess that the utilized association can be of more than one kind. So as not to be confused by large numbers we shall discuss only the most pronounced variations, and shall give only a few examples.

The association used in the substitution may be a mere sound, so that this sub-group may be analogous to word-wit in the pun. However, it is not similarity in sound of two words, but of whole sentences, characteristic combinations of words, and similar means.

For example, Lichtenberg coined the saying: *" New baths heal well,"* which immediately reminds one of the proverb, *" New brooms clean well,"* whose first and last words, as well as whose whole sentence structure, is the same as in the first saying. It has undoubtedly arisen in the witty thinker's mind as an imitation of the familiar proverb. Thus Lichtenberg's saying is an allusion to the latter. By means of this allusion something is suggested that cannot be frankly said, namely, that the efficacy of the baths taken as cures is due to other things beside the thermal springs whose attributes are the same everywhere.

The solution of the technique of another one of Lichtenberg's jokes is similar: *" The girl barely twelve modes old."* That sounds something like the chronological term *" twelve moons "* (i.e., months), and may originally have been a mistake in writing in the permissible poetical expression. But there is a good deal of sense in designating the age of a feminine creature by the changing modes instead of by the changing of moons.

The connection of similarity may even consist of a single slight modification. This technique again runs parallel with a word-technique. Both kinds of witticisms create almost the identical impression, but they are more easily distinguishable by the processes of the wit-work.

The following is an example of such a word-witticism or pun. The great singer, Mary Wilt, who was famous not merely on account of the magnitude of her voice, suffered the mortification of having a title of a play, dramatized from the well-known novel of Jules Verne, serve as an allusion to her corpulency. *" The trip around the Wilt* (world) *in eighty days."*

Or: *" Every fathom a queen,"* which is a modification of the familiar Shakespearian quotation, *" Every inch a king,"* and served as an allusion to a prominent woman who was unusually big physically. There would really be no serious objection if one should prefer to classify this witticism as a substitution for condensation with modification (cf. tête-à-bête, p. 25).

Discussing the hardships of the medical profession, namely, that physicians are obliged to read and study constantly because remedies and drugs once considered efficacious are later rejected as useless, and that despite the physician's best efforts the patient often refuses to pay for the treatment, one of the doctors present remarked: "*Yes, every drug has its day,*" to which another added, "*But not every Doc gets his pay.*" These two witty remarks are both modifications with allusion of the well-known saying, "*Every dog has his day.*" But here, too, the technique could be described as fusion with modification.

If the modification contents itself with a change in letters, allusions through modifications are barely distinguishable from condensation with substitutive formation, as shown in this example: "*Mellingitis,*" *the allusion to the dangerous disease meningitis, refers to the danger which the conservative members of a provincial borough in England thought impended if the socialist candidate Mellon were elected.*

The negative particles make very good allusions at the cost of very little changing. Heine referred to Spinoza as:

"My fellow *un*believer Spinoza."

"We, by the *Un*grace of God, Laborers, Bondsmen, Negroes, Serfs," etc., is a manifesto (which Lichtenberg quotes no further) of these unfortunates who probably have more right to that title than kings and dukes have to the unmodified one.

Omission

Finally *omission*, which is comparable to condensation without substitutive formation, is also a form of allusion. For in every allusion there is really something omitted, namely, the trend of thought that leads to the allusion. It is only a question of whether the gap, or the substitute in the wording of the allusion which partly fills in the gap, is the more obvious element. Thus we come back through a series of examples from the very clear cases of omission to those of actual allusion.

Omission without substitution is found in the following example. There lived in Vienna a clever and bellicose writer whose sharp invectives had repeatedly brought him bodily assault at the hands of the persons he assailed. During a conversation about a new misdeed by one of his habitual opponents, some one said, "*When X. hears this he will receive another box on his ear.*" The technique of this wit shows in the first place the confusion about the apparent contradiction, for it is by no means

clear to us why a box on one's ear should be
the direct result of having heard something.
The contradiction disappears if one fills in the
gap by adding to the remark: " *then he will
write such a caustic article against that person
that, etc.*" Allusions through omission and contradiction are thus the technical means of this
witticism.

Heine remarked about some one: "*He praises
himself so much that pastils for fumigation are
advancing in price.*" This omission can easily
be filled in. What has been omitted is replaced
by an inference which then strikes back as an
allusion to the same. For self-praise has always carried an evil odor with it.

Once more we encounter the two Jews in
front of the bathing establishment. "*Another
year has passed by already,*" says one with a
sigh.

These examples leave no doubt that the omission is meant as an allusion.

A still more obvious omission is contained
in the next example, which is really a genuine
and correct allusion-witticism. Subsequent to
an artists' banquet in Vienna a joke book was
given out in which, among others, the following most remarkable proverb could be read:

"*A wife is like an umbrella, at worst one may
also take a cab.*"

An umbrella does not afford enough protection from rain. The words "*at worst*" can mean only: when it is raining hard. A cab is a public conveyance. As we have to deal here with the figure of comparison, we shall put off the detailed investigation of this witticism until later on.

Heine's "Bäder von Lucca" contains a veritable wasps' nest of stinging allusions which make the most artistic use of this form of wit as polemics against the Count of Platen. Long before the reader can suspect their application, a certain theme, which does not lend itself especially to direct presentation, is preluded by allusions of the most varied material possible; e.g., in Hirsch-Hyacinth's twisting of words: You are too corpulent and I am too lean; you possess too much conceit and I the more business ability; I am a practicus and you are a diarrheticus, in fine, "You are altogether my Antipodex"—"Venus Urinia"—the thick Gudel of Dreckwall in Hamburg, etc. Then the occurrences of which the poet speaks take a turn in which it merely seems to show the impolite sportiveness of the poet, but soon it discloses the symbolic relation to the polemical intention, and in this way it also reveals itself as allusion. At last the attack against Platen bursts forth, and now the allusions to the sub-

ject of the Count's love for men seethe and
gush from each one of the sentences which
Heine directs against the talent and the character of his opponent, e.g.:

"Even if the Muses are not well disposed
to him, he has at least the genius of speech in
his power, or rather he knows how to violate
him; for he lacks the free love of this genius,
besides he must perseveringly run after this
youth, and he knows only how to grasp the
outer forms which, in spite of their beautiful
rotundity, never express anything noble."

"He has the same experience as the ostrich,
which considers itself sufficiently hidden when
it sticks its head into the sand so that only its
backside is visible. Our illustrious bird would
have done better if he had stuck his backside
into the sand, and had shown us his head."

Allusion is perhaps the commonest and most
easily employed means of wit, and is at the basis
of most of the short-lived witty productions
which we are wont to weave into our conversation. They cannot bear being separated from
their native soil nor can they exist independ-
ently. Once more we are reminded by the
process of allusion of that relationship which
has already begun to confuse our estimation of
the technique of wit. The process of allusion
is not witty in itself; there are perfectly formed

allusions which have no claims to this character.
Only those allusions which show a "witty"
element are witty, hence the characteristics of
wit, which we have followed even into its technique, again escape us.

I have sometimes called allusion "indirect expression," and now recognize that the different
kinds of allusion with representation through
the opposite, as well as the techniques still to be
mentioned, can be united into a single large
group for which "indirect expression" would
be the comprehensive name. Hence, *errors of
thought—unification—indirect representation—*
are those points of view under which we can
group the techniques of thought-wit which became known to us.

Representation Through the Minute or the Minutest Element

On continuing the investigation of our material we think we recognize a new sub-group
of indirect representation which though sharply
defined can be illustrated only by few examples.
It is that of representation through a minute
or minutest element; solving the problem by
bringing the entire character to full expression
through a minute detail. Correlating this
group with the mechanism of allusion is made

possible by looking at the triviality as connected with the thing to be presented and as a result of it. For example:

A Jew who was riding in a train had made himself very comfortable; he had unbuttoned his coat, and had put his feet on the seat, when a fashionably dressed gentleman came in. The Jew immediately put on his best behavior and assumed a modest position. The stranger turned over the pages of a book, did some calculation, and pondered a moment and suddenly addressed the Jew. "I beg your pardon, how soon will we have Yom Kippur?" (Day of Atonement). "Oh, oh!" said the Jew, and put his feet back on the seat before he answered.

It cannot be denied that this representation through something minute is allied to the tendency of economy which we found to be the final common element in the investigation of the technique of word-wit.

The following example is much similar.

The doctor who had been summoned to help the baroness in her confinement declared that the critical moment had not arrived, and proposed to the baron that they play a game of cards in the adjoining room in the meantime. After a while the doleful cry of the baroness reached the ears of the men. "Ah, mon Dieu,

que je souffre!" The husband jumped up, but
the physician stopped him saying, "*That's
nothing; let us play on."* A little while later
the woman in labor-pains was heard again:
"*My God, my God, what pains!"* "*Don't
you want to go in, Doctor?"* asked the baron.
"*By no means, it is not yet time,"* answered the
doctor. At last there rang from the adjacent
room the unmistakable cry, "*A-a-a-ai-e-e-e-e-e-
E-E-E!"* The physician then threw down the
cards and said, "*Now it's time."*

How the pain allows the original nature to
break through all the strata of education, and
how an important decision is rightly made dependent upon a seemingly inconsequential utterance—both are shown in this good joke by the
successive changes in the cries of this child-
bearing lady of quality.

Comparison

Another kind of indirect expression of which
wit makes use is *comparison,* which we have not
discussed so far because an examination of comparison touches upon new difficulties, or rather
it reveals difficulties which have made their
appearance on other occasions. We have already admitted that in many of the examples
examined we could not banish all doubts as to

whether they should really be counted as witty,
and have recognized in this uncertainty a serious
shock to the principles of our investigation.
But in no other material do I feel this uncertainty greater and nowhere does it occur more
frequently than in the case of comparison-wit.
The feeling which usually says to me—and I
dare say to a great many others under the same
conditions—this is a joke, this may be written
down as witty before even the hidden and
essential character of the wit has been uncov-
ered—this feeling I lack most. If at first I
experience no hesitation in declaring the comparison to be a witticism, then the next instant
I seem to think that the pleasure I thus found
was of a different quality than that which I am
accustomed to asci be to a joke. Also the fact
that witty comparisons but seldom can evoke
the explosive variety of laughter by which a
good joke proves itself makes it impossible for
me to cast aside the existing doubts, even when
I limit myself to the best and most effective
examples.

It is easy to demonstrate that there are some
especially good and effective examples of comparison which in no way give us the impression of witticisms. A beautiful example of this
kind which I have not yet tired of admiring,
and the impression of which still clings to me,

I shall not deny myself the pleasure of citing. It is a comparison with which Ferd. Lassalle concluded one of his famous pleas (*Die Wissenschaft und die Arbeiter*): " A man like myself who, as I explained to you, had devoted his whole life to the motto ' Die Wissenschaft und die Arbeiter ' (Science and the Workingman), would receive the same impression from a condemnation which in the couise of events confronts him *as would the chemist, absorbed in his scientific experiments, from the cracking of a retort. With a slight knitting of his brow at the resistance of the material, he would, as soon as the disturbance was quieted, calmly continue his labor and investigations.*"

One finds a rich assortment of pertinent and witty comparisons in the writings of Lichtenberg (2 B. of the Göttingen edition, 1853). I shall take the material for our investigation from that source.

" *It is almost impossible to carry the torch of truth through a crowd without singeing somebody's beard.*" This may seem witty, but on closer examination one notices that the witty effect does not come from the comparison itself but from a secondary attribute of the same. For the expression " the torch of truth " is no new comparison, but one which has been used for a long time and which has degenerated into a fixed phrase, as always happens when a comparison has the luck to be absorbed into the common usage of speech. But whereas we hardly notice the comparison in the saying, "the torch of truth," its original full force is restored it by Lichtenberg, since by building further on the comparison it results in a deduction. But the taking of blurred expressions in their full sense is already known to us as a technique of wit; it finds a place with the Manifold Application of the Same Material (p. 35). It may well be that the witty impression created by Lichtenberg's sentence is due only to its relation to this technique of wit.

The same explanation will undoubtedly hold good for another witty comparison by the same author.

"*The man was not exactly a shining light, but a great candlestick. . . . He was a professor of philosophy.*"

To call a scholar a shining light, a "*lumen mundi,*" has long ceased to be an effective comparison, whether it be originally qualified as a witticism or not. But here the comparison was freshened up and its full force was restored to it by deducting a modification from it and in this way setting up a second and new comparison. The way in which the second comparison came into existence seems to contain the condition of the witticism and not the two comparisons themselves. This would then be a case of Identical Wit Technique as in the example of the torch.

The following comparison seems witty on other but similarly classifiable grounds: " *I look upon reviews as a kind of children's disease* which more or less attacks new-born books. There are cases on record where the healthiest died of it, and the puniest have often lived through it. Many do not get it at all. Attempts have frequently been made to prevent the disease by means of *amulets of prefaces and dedications, or to color them up by personal pronunciamentos; but it does not always help.*"

The comparison of reviews with children's diseases is based in the first place upon their susceptibility to attack shortly after they have seen the light of the world. Whether this makes it witty I do not trust myself to decide. But when the comparison is continued, it is found that the later fates of the new books may be represented within the scope of the same or by means of similar comparisons. Such a continuation of a comparison is undoubtedly witty, but we know already to what technique it owes its witty flavor; it is a case of *unification* or the establishment of an unexpected association. The character of the unification, however, is not

changed by the fact that it consists here of a
relationship with the first comparison.

Doubt in Witty Comparisons

In a series of other comparisons one is
tempted to ascribe an indisputably existing
witty impression to another factor which again
in itself has nothing to do with the nature of
the comparison. These are comparisons which
are strikingly grouped, often containing a combination that sounds absurd, which comes into
existence as a result of the comparison. Most
of Lichtenberg's examples belong to this group.

"It is a pity that one cannot see the *learned
bowels* of the writers, in order to find out what
they have eaten." "*The learned bowels*" is a
confusing, really absurd attribute which is
made clear only by the comparison. How
would it be if the witty impression of this comparison should be referred entirely and fully to
the confusing character of their composition?
This would correspond to one of the means of
wit well known to us, namely, representation
through absurdity.

Lichtenberg has used the same comparison of
the imbibing of reading and educational material with the imbibing of physical nourishment.

"He thought highly of *studying in his room*

and was heartily in favor of *learned stable fodder.*"

The same absurd or at least conspicuous attributes, which as we are beginning to notice are the real carriers of the wit, mark other comparisons of the same author.

"*This is the weatherside of my moral constitution, here I can stand almost anything.*"

"Every person has also his *moral backside* which he does not show *except under the stress of necessity* and which he covers as long as possible with the *pants of good-breeding.*"

The "moral backside" is the peculiar attribute which exists as the result of a comparison. But this is followed by a continuation of the comparison with a regular play on words ("necessity") and a second, still more unusual combination ("the pants of good-breeding"), which is possibly witty in itself; for the pants become witty, as it were, because they are the pants of good-breeding. Therefore it may not take us by surprise if we get the impression of a very witty comparison; we are beginning to notice that we show a general tendency in our estimation to extend a quality to the whole thing when it clings only to one part of it. Besides, the "pants of good-breeding" remind us of a similar confusing verse of Heine.

"Until, at last, the buttons tore from the pants of my patience."

It is obvious that both of the last comparisons possess a character which one cannot find in all good, i.e., fitting, comparisons. One might say that they are in a large manner " debasing," for they place a thing of high category, an abstraction (good-breeding, patience), side by side with a thing of a very concrete nature of a very low kind (pants). Whether this peculiarity has something to do with wit we shall have to consider in another connection. Let us attempt to analyze another example in which the degrading character is exceptionally well defined. In Nestroy's farce *"Einen Jux will er sich machen,"* the clerk, Weinberl, who resolves in his imagination how he will ponder over his youth when he has some day become a well-established old merchant, says: *"When in the course of confidential conversation the ice is chopped up before the warehouse of memory; when the portal of the storehouse of antiquity is unlocked again; and when the mattings of phantasy are stocked full with wares of yore."* These are certainly comparisons of abstractions with very common, concrete things, but the witticism depends—exclusively or only partially—upon the circumstance that a clerk makes use of these comparisons which are taken from the sphere of his daily occupation. But to bring the abstract in relation to the commonplace with which he is otherwise filled is an act of *unification*. Let us revert to Lichtenberg's comparisons.

Peculiar Attributions

" *The motives for our actions may be arranged like the thirty-two winds, and their names may be classified in a similar way, e.g., Bread-bread-glory or Glory-glory-bread.*"

As so often happens ·in ʾLichtenberg's witticisms, in this case, too, the impression of appropriateness, cleverness, and ingenuity is so marked that our judgment of the character of the witty element is thereby misled. .If something witty is intermingled in such an utterance with the excellent sense, we probably are deluded into declaring the whole to be an exceptional joke. Moreover, I dare say that everything that is really witty about it results from the strangeness of the peculiar combination bread-bread-glory. Thus as far as wit is concerned it is representation through absurdity.

The peculiar combination or absurd attribution can alone be represented as a product of a comparison.

Lichtenberg says: " *A twice-sleepy woman—*

a once-sleepy church pew." Behind each one there is a comparison with a bed; in both cases there is besides the comparison also the technical factor of *allusion.* Once it is an allusion to the soporific effect of sermons, and the second time to the inexhaustible theme of sex.

Having found hitherto that a comparison as often as it appears witty owes this impression to its connection with one of the techniques of wit known to us, there are nevertheless some other examples which seem to point to the fact that a comparison as such can also be witty.

This is Lichtenberg's characteristic remark about certain odes. " They are in poetry what Jacob Böhm's immortal writings are in prose— *they are a kind of picnic in which the author supplies the words, and the readers the meaning."*

" When he *philosophizes,* he generally sheds *an agreeable moonlight* over his topics, which is in the main quite pleasant, but which does not show any one subject clearly."

Again, Heine's description: *" Her face resembled a kodex palimpsestus, where under the new block-lettered text of a church father peek forth the half-obliterated verses of an ancient Hellenic erotic poet."*

Or, the continued comparison of a very degrading tendency, in the " Bäder von Lucca."

THE TECHNIQUE OF WIT   123

"*The Catholic priest* is more like a clerk who is employed in a big business; the church, the big house at the head of which is the Pope, gives him a definite salary. He works lazily like one who is not working on his own account, he has many colleagues, and so easily remains unnoticed in the big business enterprise. He is concerned only in the credit of the house and still more in its preservation, since he would be deprived of his means of sustenance in case it went bankrupt. *The Protestant clergyman,* on the other hand, is his own boss, and carries on the religious businesses on his own account. He has no wholesale trade like his Catholic brother-tradesman, but deals merely at retail; and since he himself must understand it, he cannot be lazy. He must praise his *articles of faith* to the people and must disparage the articles of his competitors. Like a true small trader he stands in his retail store, full of envy of the industry of all large houses, particularly the large house in Rome which has so many thousand bookkeepers and packers on its payroll, and which owns factories in all four corners of the world."

In the face of this, as in many other examples, we can no longer dispute the fact that a comparison may in itself be witty, and that the witty impression need not necessarily depend

on one of the known techniques of wit. But
we are entirely in the dark as to what determines the· witty character of the comparison,
since it certainly does not cling to the similarity
as a form of expression of the thought, or to
the operation of the comparison. We can do
nothing but include comparison with the different forms of " indirect representation " which
are at the disposal of the technique of wit, and
the problem, which confronted us more distinctly in the mechanism of comparison than
in the means of wit hitherto treated, must remain unsolved. There must surely be a special
reason why the decision whether something is a
witticism or not presents more difficulties in
cases of comparison than in other forms of expression.

This gap in our understanding, however, offers no ground for complaint that our first investigation has been unsuccessful. Considering
the intimate connection which we had to be prepared to ascribe to the different types of wit,
it would have been imprudent to expect that
we could fully explain this aspect of the problem before we had cast a glance over the others.
We shall have to take up this problem at
another place.

Review of the Techniques of Wit

Are we sure that none of the possible techniques of wit has escaped our investigation? Not exactly; but by a continued examination of new material, we can convince ourselves that we have become acquainted with the most numerous and most important technical means of wit-work—at least with as much as is necessary for formulating a judgment about the nature of this psychic process. At present no such judgment exists; on the other hand, we have come into possession of important indications, from the direction of which we may expect a further explanation of the problem. The interesting processes of condensation with substitutive formation, which we have recognized as the nucleus of the technique of word-wit, directed our attention to the dream-formation in whose mechanism the identical psychic processes were discovered. Thither also we are directed by the technique of the thought-wit, namely displacement, faulty thinking, absurdity, indirect expression, and representation through the opposite—each and all are also found in the technique of dreams. The dream is indebted to displacement for its strange appearance, which hinders us from recognizing in it the continuation of our waking thoughts; the dream's use of absurdity and contradiction has cost it the dignity of a psychic product, and has misled the authors to assume that the determinants of dream-formation are: collapse of mental activity, cessation of criticism, morality, and logic. Representation through the opposite is so common in dreams that even the popular but entirely misleading books on dream interpretation usually put it to good account. Indirect expression, the substitution for the dream-thought by an allusion, by a trifle or by a symbolism analogous to comparison, is just exactly what distinguishes the manner of expression of the dream from our waking thoughts.[1] Such a far-reaching agreement as found between the means of wit-work and those of dream-work can scarcely be accidental. To show those agreements in detail and to trace their motivations will be one of our future tasks.

---

[1] Cf. my *Interpretation of Dreams*, Chap. VI, *The Dream Work*, translated by A. A. Brill, The Macmillan Co., New York, and Allen & Unwin, London.

III

NEAR the end of the preceding chapter as I was writing down Heine's comparison of the Catholic priest to an employee of a large business house, and the comparison of the Protestant divine to an independent retail dealer, I felt an inhibition which nearly prevented me from using this comparison. I said to myself that among my readers probably there would be some who hold in veneration not only religion, but also its administration and administrators. These readers might take offense at the comparison and get so wrought up about it that it would take away all interest in the investigation as to whether the comparison seemed witty in itself or was witty only through its garnishings. In other examples, e.g., the one mentioned above concerning the agreeable moonlight shed by a certain philosophy, there would be no worry that for some readers it might be a disturbing influence in our investi-

---

[1] The word tendency encountered hereafter in the expression " Tendency-Wit " (Tendenz Witz) is used adjectively in the same sense as in the familiar phrase " Tendency Play."

gation. Even the most religious person would remain in the right mood to form a judgment about our problem.

It is easy to guess the character of the witticism by the kind of reaction that wit exerts on the hearer. Sometimes wit is wit for its own sake and serves no other particular purpose; then again, it places itself at the service of such a purpose, i.e., it becomes purposive. Only that form of wit which has such a tendency runs the risk of ruffling people who do not wish to hear it.

Theo. Vischer called wit without a tendency " *abstract* " wit, I prefer to call it " *harmless* " wit.

As we have already classified wit according to the material touched by its technique into word- and thought-wit, it is incumbent upon us to investigate the relation of this classification to the one just put forward. Word- and thought-wit on the one hand, and abstract- and tendency-wit on the other hand, bear no relation of dependence to each other; they are two entirely independent classifications of witty productions. Perhaps some one may have gotten the impression that harmless witticisms are preponderately word-witticisms, whereas the complicated techniques of thought-witticisms are mostly made to serve strong tendencies. There

are harmless witticisms that operate through
play on words and sound similarity, and just as
harmless ones which make use of all means of
thought-wit. Nor is it less easy to prove that
tendency-wit as far as technique is concerned
may be merely the wit of words. Thus, for example, witticisms that "*play*" with proper
names often show an insulting and offending
tendency, and yet they, too, belong to word-wit.
Again, the most harmless of all jests are word-
witticisms. Examples of this nature are the
popular "shake-up" rhymes (Schüttelreime)
in which the technique is represented through
the manifold application of the same material
with a very peculiar modification:
"Having been forsaken by *Dame Luck,* he
degenerated into a *Lame Duck.*"
Let us hope that no one will deny that the
pleasure experienced in this kind of otherwise
unpretentious rhyming is of the same nature as
the one by which we recognize wit.

Good examples of abstract or harmless
thought-witticisms abound in Lichtenberg's comparisons with which we have already become acquainted. I add a few more. "*They sent a
small Octavo to the University of Göttingen;
and received back in body and soul a quarto*"
(a fourth-form boy).

"*In order to erect this building well, one*

*must lay above all things a good foundation,
and I know of no firmer than by laying immediately over every pro-layer a contra-layer."*

" *One man begets the thought, the second
acts as its godfather, the third begets children
by it, the fourth visits it on its death-bed, and
the fifth buries it* " (comparison with unification).

" *Not only did he disbelieve in ghosts, but he
was not ever afraid of them.*" The witticism in
this case lies exclusively in the absurd representation which puts what is usually considered
less important in the comparative and what is
considered more important in the positive degree. If we divest it of its dress it says: it is
much easier to use our reason and make light
of the fear of ghosts than to defend ourselves
against this fear when the occasion presents itself. But this rendering is no longer witty; it
is merely a correct and still too little respected
psychological fact suggesting what Lessing expresses in his well-known words:

" Not all are free who mock their chains."

Harmless and Tendency Wit

I shall take the opportunity presented here
of clearing up what may still lead to a possible

misunderstanding. "Harmless" or "abstract" wit should in no way convey the same meaning as "shallow" or "poor" wit. It is meant only to designate the opposite of the "tendency" wit to be described later. As shown in the aforementioned examples, a harmless jest, i.e., a witticism without a tendency, can also be very rich in content and express something worth while. The quality of a witticism, however, is independent of the wit and represents the quality of the thought which is here expressed wittily by means of a special contrivance. To be sure, just as watch-makers are wont to enclose very good works in valuable cases, so it may likewise happen with wit that the best witty activities are used to invest the richest thoughts.

Now, if we pay strict attention to the distinction between thought-content and the witty wording of thought-wit, we arrive at an insight which may clear up much uncertainty in our judgment of wit. For it turns out—astonishing as it may seem—that our enjoyment of a witticism is supplied by the combined impression of content and wit-activity, and that one of the factors is likely to deceive us about the extent of the other. It is only the reduction of the witticism that lays bare to us our mistaken judgment.

The same thing applies to word-wit. When we hear that *"experience consists simply of experiencing what one wishes he had not experienced,"* we are puzzled, and believe that we have learnt a new truth; it takes some time before we recognize in this disguise the platitude, "adversity is the school of wisdom" (K. Fischer). The excellent wit-activity which seeks to define "experience" by the almost exclusive use of the word "experience" deceives us so completely that we overestimate the content of the sentence. The same thing happens in many similar cases and also in Lichtenberg's unification-witticism about January (p. 89), which expresses nothing but what we already know, namely, that New Year's wishes are as seldom realized as other wishes.

We find the contrary true of other witticisms, in which obviously what is striking and correct in the thought captivates us, so that we call the saying an excellent witticism, whereas it is only the thought that is brilliant while the wit-activity is often weak. It is especially true of Lichtenberg's wit that the path of the thought is often of more value than its witty expression, though we unjustly extend the value of the former to the latter. Thus the remark about the "torch of truth" (p. 115) is hardly a witty comparison, but it is so striking that we are inclined to lay stress on the sentence as exceptionally witty.

Lichtenberg's witticisms are above all remarkable for their thought-content and their certainty of hitting the mark. Goethe has rightly remarked about this author that his witty and jocose thoughts positively conceal problems. Or perhaps it may be more correct to say that they touch upon the solutions of problems. When, for example, he presents as a witty thought:

" He always read *Agamemnon* instead of the German word *angenommen,* so thoroughly had he read Homer " (technically this is absurdity plus sound similarity of words). Thus he discovered nothing less than the secret of mistakes in reading.[1] The following joke, whose technique (p. 78) seemed to us quite unsatisfactory, is of a similar nature.

" *He was surprised that there were two holes cut in the pelts of cats just where the eyes were located.*" The stupidity here exhibited is only seemingly so; in reality this ingenuous remark conceals the great problem of teleology in the structure of animals; it is not at all so self-evident that the eyelid cleft opens just where the

---

[1] Cf. my *Psychopathology of Everyday Life,* translated by A. A. Brill, The Macmillan Co., New York, and T. Fisher Unwin, London.

cornea is exposed, until the science of evolution explains to us this coincidence.

Let us bear in mind that a witty sentence gave us a general impression in which we were unable to distinguish the amount of thought-content from the amount of wit-work; perhaps even a more significant parallel to it will be found later.

Pleasure Results from the Technique

For our theoretical explanation of the nature of wit, harmless wit must be of greater value to us than tendency-wit and shallow wit more than profound wit. Harmless and shallow plays on words present to us the problem of wit in its purest form, because of the good sense therein and because there is no purposive factor nor underlying philosophy to confuse the judgment. With such material our understanding can make further progress.

At the end of a dinner to which I had been invited, a pastry called Roulard was served; it was a culinary accomplishment which presupposed a good deal of skill on the part of the cook. " Is it home-made? " asked one of the guests. " Oh, yes," replied the host, " it is a Home-Roulard " (Home Rule).

This time we shall not investigate the technique of this witticism, but shall center our attention upon another, and that one the most important factor. As I remember, this improvised joke delighted all the guests and made us laugh. In this case, as in countless others, the feeling of pleasure of the hearer cannot have originated from any purposive element nor the thought-content of the wit; so we are forced to connect the feeling of pleasure with the technique of wit. The technical means of wit which we have described, such as condensation, displacement, indirect expression, etc., have therefore the faculty to produce a feeling of pleasure in the hearer, although we cannot as yet see how they acquired that faculty. By such easy stages we get the second axiom for the explanation of wit; the first one (p. 17) states that the character of wit depends upon the mode of expression. Let us remember also that the second axiom has really taught us nothing new. It merely isolates a fact that was already contained in a discovery which we made before. For we recall that whenever it was possible to reduce the wit by substituting for its verbal expression another set of words, at the same time carefully retaining the sense, it not only eliminated the witty character but also the laughableness (*Lacheffekt*) that constitutes the pleasure of wit.

At present we cannot go further without first coming to an understanding with our philosophical authorities.

The philosophers who adjudge wit to be a part of the comic and deal with the latter itself in the field of æsthetics, characterize the æsthetic presentation by the following conditions: that we are not thereby interested in or about the objects, that we do not need these objects to satisfy our great wants in life, but that we are satisfied with the mere contemplation of the same, and with the pleasure of the thought itself. " This pleasure, this mode of conception is purely æsthetical, it depends entirely on itself, its end is only itself and it fulfills no other end in life " (K. Fischer, p. 68).

We scarcely venture a contradiction to K. Fischer's words—perhaps we merely translate his thoughts into our own mode of expression —when we insist that the witty activity is, after all, not to be designated as aimless or purposeless, since it has for its aim the evocation of pleasure in the hearer. I doubt whether we are able to undertake anything which has no object in view. When we do not use our psychic apparatus for the fulfillment of one of our indispensable gratifications, we let it work for pleasure, and we seek to derive pleasure from its own activity. I suspect that this is really the condition which underlies all æsthetic thinking, but I know too little about æsthetics to be willing to support this theory. About wit, however, I can assert, on the strength of the two impressions gained before, that it is an activity whose purpose is to derive pleasure—be it intellectual or otherwise—from the psychic processes. To be sure, there are other activities which accomplish the same thing. They may be differentiated from each by the sphere of psychic activity from which they wish to derive pleasure, or perhaps by the methods which they use in accomplishing this. At present we cannot decide this, but we firmly maintain that at last we have established a connection between the technique of wit partly controlled by the tendency to economize (p. 53) and the production of pleasure.

But before we proceed to solve the riddle of how the technical means of wit-work can produce pleasure in the hearer, we wish to mention that, for the sake of simplicity and more lucidity, we have altogether put out of the way all tendency witticisms. Still we must attempt to explain what the tendencies of wit are and in what manner wit makes use of these tendencies.

Hostile and Obscene Wit

We are taught above all by an observation not to put aside the tendency-wit when we are investigating the origin of the pleasure in wit. The pleasurable effect of harmless wit is usually of a moderate nature; all that it can be expected to produce in the hearer is a distinct feeling of satisfaction and a slight ripple of laughter; and as we have shown by fitting examples (p. 132) at least a part of this effect is due to the thought-content. The sudden irresistible outburst of laughter evoked by the tendency-wit rarely follows the wit without a tendency. As the technique may be identical in both, it is fair to assume that by virtue of its purpose, the tendency-wit has at its disposal sources of pleasure to which harmless wit has no access.

It is now easy to survey wit-tendencies. Wherever wit is not a means to its end, i. e., harmless, it puts itself in the service of but two tendencies which may themselves be united under one viewpoint; it is either *hostile* wit serving as an aggression, satire, or defense, or it is *obscene* wit serving as a sexual exhibition. Again it is to be observed that the technical form of wit—be it a word- or thought-witticism—bears no relation to these two tendencies.

It is a much more complicated matter to show in what way wit serves these tendencies. In this investigation I wish to present first not the hostile but the exhibition wit. The latter has indeed very seldom been deemed worthy of an investigation, as if an aversion had transferred itself here from the material to the subject; however, we shall not allow ourselves to be misled thereby, for we shall soon touch upon a detail in wit which promises to throw light on more than one obscure point.

We all know what is meant by a " smutty " joke. It is the intentional bringing into prominence of sexual facts or relations through speech. However, this definition is no sounder than other definitions. A lecture on the anatomy of the sexual organs or on the physiology of reproduction need not, in spite of this definition, have anything in common with an obscenity. It must be added that the smutty joke is directed toward a certain person who excites one sexually, and who becomes cognizant of the speaker's excitement by listening to the smutty joke, and thereby in turn becomes sexually excited. Instead of becoming sexually excited the listener may react with shame and embarrassment, which merely signifies a reaction against the excitement and indirectly an admission of the same. The smutty joke was originally directed against the woman and is comparable to an attempt at seduction. If a man tells or listens to obscene jokes in male society, the original situation, which cannot be realized on account of social inhibitions, is thereby also represented. Whoever laughs at a smutty joke does the same as the spectator who laughs at a sexual aggression.

The sexual element which is at the basis of the obscene joke comprises more than that which is peculiar to both sexes, and goes beyond that which is common to both sexes, it is connected with all these things that cause shame, and includes the whole domain of the excrementitious. However, this was the sexual domain of childhood, where the imagination fancied a cloaca, so to speak, within which the sexual elements were either badly or not at all differentiated from the excrementitious.[1] In the whole mental domain of the psychology of the neuroses, the sexual still includes the excrementitious, and it is understood in the old, infantile sense..

The smutty joke is like the denudation of a person of the opposite sex toward whom the joke is directed. Through the utterance of ob-

[1] Cf. *Three Contributions to the Theory of Sex*, 2nd Ed., 1916, translated by A. A. Brill, Monograph Series, *Journal of Nervous and Mental Diseases*.

scene words the person attacked is forced to picture the parts of the body in question, or the sexual act, and is shown that the aggressor himself pictures the same thing. There is no doubt that the original motive of the smutty joke was the pleasure of seeing the sexual displayed.

It will only help to clarify the subject if here we go back to the fundamentals. One of the primitive components of our libido is the desire to see the sexual exposed. Perhaps this itself is a development—a substitution for the desire to touch which is assumed to be the primary pleasure. As it often happens, the desire to see has here also replaced the desire to touch.[1] The libido for looking and touching is found in every person in two forms, active and passive, or masculine and feminine; and in accordance with the preponderance of sex characteristics it develops preponderately in one or the other direction. In young children one can readily observe the desire to exhibit themselves nude. If the germ of this desire does not experience the usual fate of being covered up and repressed, it develops into a mania for exhibitionism, a familiar perversion among grown-up men. In women the passive desire to exhibit

[1] Moll's *Kontrektationstrieb* (Untersuchungen über die Libido sexualies, 1898).

is almost regularly covered by the masked re-action of sexual modesty; despite this, however, remnants of this desire may always be seen in women's dress. I need only mention how flexible and variable convention and circumstances make that remaining portion of exhibitionism still allowed to women.

The Transformation of the Obscenity into Obscene Wit

In the case of men a great part of this striving to exhibit remains as a part of the libido and serves to initiate the sexual .act. If this striving asserts itself on first meeting the woman it must make use of speech for two motives. First, in order to make itself known to the woman; and secondly, because the awakening of the imagination through speech puts the woman herself in a corresponding excitement and awakens in her the desire to passive exhibitionism. This speech of courtship is not yet smutty, but may pass over into the same. Wherever the yieldingness of the woman manifests itself quickly, smutty speech is short-lived, for it gives way to the sexual act. It is different if the rapid yielding of the woman cannot be counted upon, but instead there appears the defense reaction. In that case the sexually exciting speech changes into obscene wit as its own end; as the sexual aggression is inhibited in its progress towards the act, it lingers at the evocation of the excitement and derives pleasure from the indications of the same in the woman. In this process the aggression changes its character in the same way as any libidinous impulse confronted by a hindrance; it becomes distinctly hostile and cruel, and utilizes the sadistical components of the sexual impulse against the hindrance.

Thus the unyieldingness of the woman is therefore the next condition for the development of smutty wit; to be sure, this resistance must be of the kind to indicate merely a deferment and make it appear that further efforts will not be in vain. The ideal case of such resistance on the part of the woman usually results from the simultaneous presence of another man, a third person, whose presence almost excludes the immediate yielding of the woman. This third person soon becomes of the greatest importance for the development of the smutty wit, but next to him the presence of the woman must be taken account of. Among rural people or in the ordinary hostelry one can observe that not till the waitress or the hostess approaches the guests does the obscene wit come out; in a higher order of society just the opposite happens, here the presence of a woman puts an end to smutty talk. The men reserve this kind of conversation, which originally presupposed the presence of bashful women, until they are alone, " by themselves." Thus gradually the spectator, now turned the listener, takes the place of the woman as the object of the smutty joke, and through such a change the smutty joke already approaches the character of wit.

Henceforth our attention may be centered upon two factors, first upon the rôle that the third person—the listener—plays, and secondly, upon the intrinsic conditions of the smutty joke itself.

Tendency-wit usually requires three persons. Besides the one who makes the wit there is a second person who is taken as the object of the hostile or sexual aggression, and a third person in whom the purpose of the wit to produce pleasure is fulfilled. We shall later on inquire into the deeper motive of this relationship, for the present we shall adhere to the fact which states that it is not the maker of the wit who laughs about it and enjoys its pleasurable effect, but it is the idle listener who does. The same relationship exists among the three persons connected with the smutty joke. The process may be described as follows: As soon as the libidinous impulse of the first person, to satisfy himself through the woman, is blocked, he immediately develops a hostile attitude towards this second person and takes the originally intruding third person as his confederate. Through the obscene speech of the first person the woman is exposed before the third person, who as a listener is fascinated by the easy gratification of his own libido.

It is curious that common people so thoroughly enjoy such smutty talk, and that it is a never-lacking activity of cheerful humor. It is also worthy of notice that in this complicated process which shows so many characteristics of tendency-wit, no formal demands, such as characterize wit, are made upon "smutty wit." The unveiled nudity affords pleasure to the first and makes the third person laugh.

Not until we come to the refined and cultured does the formal determination of wit arise. The obscenity becomes witty and is tolerated only if it is witty. The technical means of which it mostly makes use is allusion, i.e., substitution through a trifle, something remotely related, which the listener reconstructs in his imagination as a full-fledged and direct obscenity. The greater the disproportion between what is directly offered in the obscenity and what is necessarily aroused by it in the mind of the listener, the finer is the witticism and the higher it may venture in good society. Besides the coarse and delicate allusions, the witty obscenity also utilizes all other means of word- and thought-wit, as can be easily demonstrated by examples.

The Function of Wit in the Service of the Tendency

It now becomes comprehensible what wit accomplishes through this service of its tendency. It makes possible the gratification of a craving (lewd or hostile) despite a hindrance which stands in the way; it eludes the hindrance and so derives pleasure from a source that has become inaccessible on account of the hindrance. The hindrance in the way is really nothing more than the higher degree of culture and education which correspondingly increases the inability of the woman to tolerate the stark sex. The woman thought of as present in the final situation is still considered present, or her influence acts as a deterrent to the men even in her absence. One often notices how cultured men are influenced by the company of girls of a lower station in life to change witty obscenities to broad smut.

The power which renders it difficult or im-

possible for the woman, and in a lesser degree
for the man, to enjoy unveiled obscenities we
call "repression," and we recognize in it the
same psychic process which keeps from consciousness in severe nervous attacks whole com-
plexes of emotions with their resultant affects,
and has shown itself to be the principal factor
in the causation of the so-called psychoneuroses.
We acknowledge to culture and higher civilization an important influence in the development of repressions, and assume that under
these conditions there has come about a change
in our psychic organization which may also
have been brought along as an inherited disposition. In consequence of it, what was once
accepted as pleasureful is now counted unac-
ceptable and is rejected by means of all the
psychic forces. Owing to the repression
brought about by civilization many primary
pleasures are now disapproved by the censor
and lost. But the human psyche finds renunciation very difficult; hence we discover that
tendency-wit furnishes us with a means to make
the renunciation retrogressive and thus to regain what has been lost. When we laugh over
a delicately obscene witticism, we laugh at the
identical thing which causes laughter in the ill-
bred man when he hears a coarse, obscene joke;
in both cases the pleasure comes from the

same source. The coarse, obscene joke, however, could not incite us to laughter, because it would cause us shame or would seem to us disgusting; we can laugh only when wit comes to our aid.

What we had presumed in the beginning seems to have been confirmed, namely, that tendency-wit has access to other sources of pleasure than harmless wit, in which all the pleasure is somehow dependent upon the technique. We can also reiterate that owing to our feelings we are in no position to distinguish in tendency-wit what part of the pleasure originates from the technique and what part from the tendency. *Strictly speaking, we do not know what we are laughing about.* In all obscene jokes we succumb to striking mistakes of judgment about the "goodness" of the joke as far as it depends upon formal conditions; the technique of these jokes is often very poor while their laughing effect is enormous.

Invectives Made Possible Through Wit

We next wish to determine whether the rôle of wit in the service of the hostile tendency is the same.

Right from the start we meet with similar

conditions. Since our individual childhood and the childhood of human civilization, our hostile impulses towards our fellow-beings have been subjected to the same restrictions and the same progressive repressions as our sexual strivings. We have not yet progressed so far as to love our enemies, or to extend to them our left cheek after we are smitten on the right. Furthermore, all moral codes about the subjection of active hatred bear even to-day the clearest indications that they were originally meant for a small community of clansmen. As we all may consider ourselves members of some nation, we permit ourselves for the most part to forget these restrictions in matters touching a foreign people. But within our own circles we have nevertheless made progress in the mastery of hostile emotions. Lichtenberg drastically puts it when he says: " Where nowadays one says, ' I beg your pardon,' formerly one had recourse to a cuff on the ear." Violent hostility, no longer tolerated by law, has been replaced by verbal invectives, and the better understanding of the concatenation of human emotions robs us, through its consequential " *Tout comprendre c'est tout pardonner,*" more and more of the capacity to become angry at our fellowman who is in our way. Having been endowed with a strong hostile disposition

in our childhood, higher personal civilization
teaches us later that it is undignified to use
abusive language; even where combat is still
permitted, the number of things which may be
used as means of combat has been markedly
restricted. Society, as the third and dispassion-
ate party in the combat to whose interest it
is to safeguard personal safety, prevents us
from expressing our hostile feelings in action;
and hence, as in sexual aggression, there has
developed a new technique of invectives, the
aim of which is to enlist this third person
against our enemy. By belittling and hum-
bling our enemy, by scorning and ridiculing
him, we indirectly obtain the pleasure of his
defeat by the laughter of the third person,
the inactive spectator.

We are now prepared for the rôle that wit
plays in hostile aggression. Wit permits us
to make our enemy ridiculous through that
which we could not utter loudly or consciously
on account of existing hindrances; in other
words, *wit affords us the means of surmounting restrictions and of opening up otherwise
inaccessible pleasure sources.* Moreover, the
listener will be induced by the gain in pleasure to take our part, even if he is not altogether convinced,—just as we on other occasions, when fascinated by harmless witticism,

were wont to overestimate the substance of the sentence wittily expressed. "To prejudice the laughter in one's own favor" is a completely pertinent saying in the German language.

One may recall Mr. N.'s witticism given in the last chapter (p. 28). It is of an insulting nature, as if the author wished to shout loudly: But the minister of agriculture is himself an ox! But he, as a man of culture, could not put his opinion in this form. He therefore appealed to wit which assured his opinion a reception at the hands of the listeners which, in spite of its amount of truth, never would have been received if in an unwitty form. Brill cites an excellent example of a similar kind: *Wendell Phillips, according to a recent biography by Dr. Lorenzo Sears, was on one occasion lecturing in Ohio, and while on a railroad journey going to keep one of his appointments met in the car a number of clergymen returning from some sort of convention. One of the ministers, feeling called upon to approach Mr. Phillips, asked him, "Are you Mr. Phillips?" "I am, sir." "Are you trying to free the niggers?" "Yes, sir; I am an abolitionist." "Well, why do you preach your doctrines up here? Why don't you go over into Kentucky?" "Excuse me, are you a preacher?"* *"I am, sir."* *"Are you trying to save souls from hell?"* *"Yes, sir, that's my business."* *"Well, why don't you go there?"* The assailant hurried into the smoker amid a roar of unsanctified laughter. This anecdote nicely illustrates the tendency-wit in the service of hostile aggression. The minister's behavior was offensive and irritating, yet Wendell Phillips as a man of culture could not defend himself in the same manner as a common, ill-bred person would have done, and as his inner feelings must have prompted him to do. The only alternative under the circumstances would have been to take the affront in silence, had not wit showed him the way, and enabled him by the technical means of unification to turn the tables on his assailant. He not only belittled him and turned him into ridicule, but by his clever retort, "Well, why don't you go there?" fascinated the other clergymen, and thus brought them to his side.

Although the hindrance to the aggression which the wit helped to elude was in these cases of an inner nature—the æsthetic resistance against insulting—it may at other times be of a purely outer nature. So it was in the case when Serenissimus asked the stranger who had a striking resemblance to himself: "Was your mother ever in my home?"

and he received the ready reply, "No, but my father was." The stranger would certainly have felled the imprudent inquirer who dared to make an ignominious allusion to the memory of his mother; but this imprudent person was Serenissimus, who may not be felled and not even insulted unless one wishes to pay for this revenge with his life. The only thing left was to swallow the insult in silence; but luckily wit pointed out the way of requiting the insult without personally imperiling one's self. It was accomplished simply by treating the allusion with the technical means of unification and employing it against the aggressor. The impression of wit is here so thoroughly determined by the tendency that in view of the witty rejoinder we are inclined to forget that the aggressor's inquiry is itself made witty by allusion.

Rebellion Against Authority Through Wit

The prevention of abuse or insulting retorts through outer circumstances is so often the case that tendency-wit is used with special preference as a weapon of attack or criticism of superiors who claim to be an authority. Wit then serves as a resistance against such authority and as an escape from its pressure,

In this factor, too, lies the charm of caricature, at which we laugh even if it is badly done
simply because we consider its resistance to
authority a great merit.

If we keep in mind that tendency-wit is so
well adapted as a weapon of attack upon what
is great, dignified, and mighty, that which is
shielded by internal hindrances or external
circumstance against direct disparagement, we
are forced to a special conception of certain
groups of witticisms which seem to occupy
themselves with inferior and powerless persons.
I am referring to the marriage-agent stories,—
with a few of which we have become familiar
in the investigation of the manifold techniques
of thought-wit. In some of these examples,
" But she is deaf, too! " and " Who in the world
would ever lend these people anything! " the
agent was derided as a careless and thoughtless
person who becomes comical because the truth
escapes his lips automatically, as it were. But
does on the one hand what we have learned
about the nature of tendency-wit, and on the
other hand the amount of satisfaction in these
stories, harmonize with the misery of the persons at whom the joke seems to be pointed?
Are these worthy opponents of the wit? Or,
is it not more plausible to suppose that the
wit puts the agent in the foreground only in

order to strike at something more important; does it, as the saying goes, strike the saddle pack, when it is meant for the mule? This conception can really not be rejected.

The above-mentioned interpretation of the marriage-agent stories admits of a continuation. It is true that I need not enter into them, that I can content myself with seeing the farcical in these stories, and can dispute their witty character. However, such subjective determination of wit actually exists. We have now become cognizant of it and shall later on have to investigate it. It means that only that is a witticism which I wish to consider as such. What may be wit to me, may be only an amusing story to another. But if a witticism admits of doubt, that can be due only to the fact that it is possessed of a show-side,—in our examples it happens to be a façade of the comic,—upon which one may be satisfied to bestow a single glance while another may attempt to peep behind. We also suspect that this façade is intended to dazzle the prying glance which is to say that such stories have something to conceal.

At all events, if our marriage-agent stories are witticisms at all, they are all the better witticisms because, thanks to their façade, they are in a position to conceal not only what they have to say but also that they have something —forbidden—to say. But the continuation of the interpretation, which reveals this hidden part and shows that these stories having a comical façade are tendency-witticisms, would be as follows: Every one who allows the truth to escape his lips in an unguarded moment is really pleased to have rid himself of this thought. This is a correct and far-reaching psychological insight. Without the inner assent no one would allow himself to be overpowered by the automatism which here brings the truth to light.[1] The marriage agent is thus transformed from a ludicrous personage into an object deserving of pity and sympathy. How blest must be the man, able at last to un-burden himself of the weight of dissimulation, if he immediately seizes the first opportunity to shout out the last fragment of truth! As soon as he sees that his case is lost, that the prospective bride does not suit the young man, he gladly betrays the secret that the girl has still another blemish which the young man had overlooked, or he makes use of the chance to present a conclusive argument in detail in order to express his contempt for the people

---

[1] It is the same mechanism that controls " slips of the tongue " and other phenomena of self-betrayal. Cf. *The Psychopathology of Everyday Life.*

who employ him: "Who in the world would ever lend these people anything!" The ludicrousness of the whole thing now reverts upon the parents,—hardly mentioned in the story,—who consider such deceptions justified to clutch a man for their daughter; it also reflects upon the wretched state of the girls who get married through such contrivances, and upon the want of dignity of the marriage contracted after such preliminaries. The agent is the right person to express such criticisms, for he is best acquainted with these abuses; but he may not raise his voice, because he is a poor man whose livelihood depends altogether on turning these abuses to his advantage. But the same conflict is found in the national spirit which has given rise to these and similar stories; for he is aware that the holiness of wedlock suffers severely by reference to some of the methods of marriage-making.

We recall also the observation made during the investigation of wit-technique, namely, that absurdity in wit frequently stands for derision and criticism in the thought behind the witticism, wherein the wit-work follows the dream-work. This state of affairs, we find, is here once more confirmed. That the derision and criticism are not aimed at the agent, who appears in the former examples only as the whip-

ping boy of the joke, is shown by another series
in which the agent, on the contrary, is pictured
as a superior person whose dialectics are a
match for any difficulty. They are stories
whose façades are logical instead of comical—
they are sophistic thought-witticisms. In one
of them (p. 83) the agent knows how to circumvent the limping of the bride by stating
that in her case it is at least " a finished job ";
another woman with straight limbs would be
in constant danger of falling and breaking
a leg, which would be followed by sickness,
pains, and doctor's fees—all of which can be
avoided by marrying the one already limping.
Again in another example (p. 81) the agent
is clever enough to refute by good arguments each of the whole series of the suitor's
objections against the bride; only to the
last, which cannot be glossed over, he re-
joins, " Do you expect her to have no blemishes at all? " as if the other objections had
not left behind an important remnant. It is
not difficult to pick out the weak points of the
arguments in both examples, a thing which we
have done during the investigation of the technique. But now something else interests us.
If the agent's speech is endowed with such a
strong semblance of logic, which on more careful examination proves to be merely a sem-

blance, then the truth must be lurking in the fact that the witticism adjudges the agent to be right. The thought does not dare to admit that he is right in all seriousness, and replaces it by the semblance which the wit brings forth; but here, as it often happens, the jest betrays the seriousness of it. We shall not err if we assume that all stories with logical façades really mean what they assert even if these assertions are deliberately falsely motivated. Only this use of sophism for the veiled presentation of the truth endows it with the character of wit, which is mainly dependent upon tendency. What these two stories wish to indicate is that the suitor really makes himself ridiculous when he collects together so sedulously the individual charms of the bride which are transient after all, and when he forgets at the same time that he must be prepared to take as his wife a human being with inevitable faults; whereas, the only virtue which might make tolerable marriage with the more or less imperfect personality of the woman,—mutual attachment and willingness for affectionate adaptation,—is not once mentioned in the whole affair.

Ridicule of the suitor as seen in these examples in which the agent quite correctly assumes the rôle of superiority, is much more clearly depicted in other examples. The more pointed the stories, the less wit-technique they contain; they are, as it were, merely border-line cases of wit with whose technique they have only the façade-formation in common. However, in view of the same tendency and the concealment of the same behind the façade, they obtain the full effect of wit. The poverty of technical means makes it clear also that many witticisms of that kind cannot dispense with the comic element of jargon which acts similarly to wit-technique without great sacrifices.

The following is such a story, which with all the force of tendency-wit obviates all traces of that technique. *The agent asks: "What are you looking for in your bride?" The reply is: "She must be pretty, she must be rich, and she must be cultured." "Very well," was the agent's rejoinder. "But what you want will make three matches."* Here the reproach is no longer embodied in wit, but is made directly to the man.

In all the preceding examples the veiled aggression was still directed against persons; in the marriage-agent jokes it is directed against all the parties involved in the betrothal—the bridegroom, bride, and her parents. The object of attack by wit may equally well be institutions, persons, in so far as they may act as agents of these, moral or religious precepts, or even philosophies of life which enjoy so much respect that they can be challenged in no other way than under the guise of a witticism, and one that is veiled by a façade at that. No matter how few the themes upon which tendency-wit may play, its forms and investments are manifold. I believe that we shall do well to designate this species of tendency-wit by a special name. To decide what name will be appropriate is possible only after analyzing a few examples of this kind.

The Witty Cynicism

I recall the two little stories about the impecunious gourmand who was caught eating " salmon with mayonnaise," and about the tippling tutor; these witty stories, which we have learned to regard as sophistical displacement-wit, I shall continue to analyze. We have learned since then that when the semblance of logic is attached to the façade of a story, the actual thought is as follows: The man is right; but on account of the opposing contradiction, I did not dare to admit the fact except for one point in which his error is easily demonstrable. The " point " chosen is the correct compromise between his right and his wrong; this is really no decision, but bespeaks the conflict within ourselves. Both stories are simply epicurean. They say, Yes, the man is right; nothing is greater than pleasure, and it is fairly immaterial in what manner one procures it. This sounds frightfully immoral, and perhaps it is, but fundamentally it is nothing more than the " *Carpe diem* " of the poet who refers to the uncertainty of life and the bareness of virtuous renunciation. If we are repelled by the idea that the man in the joke about " salmon with mayonnaise " is in the right, then it is merely due to the fact that it illustrates the sound sense of the man in indulging himself—an indulgence which seems to us wholly unnecessary. In reality each one of us has experienced hours and times during which he has admitted the justice of this philosophy of life and has reproached our system of morality for knowing only how to make claims upon us without reimbursing us. Since we no longer lend credence to the idea of a hereafter in which all former renunciations are supposed to be rewarded by gratification—(there are very few pious persons if one makes renunciation the password of faith)— " *Carpe diem* " becomes the first admonition. I am quite ready to postpone the gratification, but how do I know whether I shall still be alive to-morrow?

"Di doman' non c'e certezza." [1]

I am quite willing to give up all the paths to gratification interdicted by society, but am I sure that society will reward me for this renunciation by opening for me—even after a certain delay—one of the permitted paths? One can plainly tell what these witticisms whisper, namely, that the wishes and desires of man have a right to make themselves perceptible next to our pretentious and inconsiderate morality. And in our times it has been said in emphatic and striking terms that this morality is merely the selfish precept of the few rich and mighty who can gratify their desires at any time without deferment. As long as the art of healing has not succeeded in safeguarding our lives, and as long as the social organizations do not do more towards making conditions more agreeable, just so long cannot the voice within us which is striving against the demands of morality, be stifled. Every honest person finally makes this admission—at least to himself. The decision in this conflict is possible only through the roundabout way of a new understanding. One must be able to knit

[1] "There is nothing certain about to-morrow," Lorenzo dei Medici.

one's life so closely to that of others, and to form such an intimate identification with others, that the shortening of one's own term of life becomes surmountable; one should not unlawfully fulfill the demands of one's own needs, but should leave them unfulfilled, because only the continuance of so many unfulfilled demands can develop the power to recast the social order. But not all personal needs allow themselves to be displaced in such a manner and transferred to others, nor is there a universal and definite solution of the conflict.

We now know how to designate the witticisms just discussed; they are cynical witticisms, and what they conceal are cynicisms.

Among the institutions which cynical wit is wont to attack there is none more important and more completely protected by moral precepts, and yet more inviting of attack, than the institution of marriage. Most of the cynical jokes are directed against it. For no demand is more personal than that made upon sexual freedom, and nowhere has civilization attempted to exert a more stringent suppression than in the realm of sexuality. For our purposes a single example suffices: the "Entries in the Album of Prince Carnival" mentioned on page 108.

A wife is like an umbrella, at worst one may always take a cab."

We have already elucidated the complicated technique of this example; it is a puzzling and seemingly impossible comparison which however, as we now see, is not in itself witty; it shows besides an allusion (cab=public conveyance), and as the strongest technical means it also shows an omission which serves to make it still more unintelligible. The comparison may be worked out in the following manner. A man marries in order to guard himself against the temptations of sensuality, but it then turns out that after all marriage affords no gratification for one of stronger needs, just as one takes along an umbrella for protection against rain only to get wet in spite of it. In both cases one must search for better protection; in one case one must take a public cab, in the other women procurable for money. Now the wit has almost entirely been replaced by cynicism. That marriage is not the organization which can satisfy a man's sexuality, one does not dare to say loudly and frankly unless indeed it be one like Christian v. Ehrenfels,[1] who is forced to it by the love of truth and the zeal of reform. The strength of this witticism

[1] See his essays in the *Politisch-anthropologischen Revue*, II, 1903.

lies in the fact that it has expressed the thought even though it had to be done through all sorts of roundabout ways.

Cynical Witticisms and Self-criticism

A particularly favorable case for tendency-wit results if the intended criticism of the inner resistance is directed against one's own person, or, more carefully expressed, against a person in whom one takes interest, that is, a composite personality such as one's own people. This determination of self-criticism may make clear why it is that a number of the most excellent jokes of which we have shown here many specimens should have sprung into existence from the soil of Jewish national life. They are stories which were invented by Jews themselves and which are directed against Jewish peculiarities. The Jewish jokes made up by non-Jews are nearly all brutal buffooneries in which the wit is spared by the fact that the Jew appears as a comic figure to a stranger. The Jewish jokes which originate with Jews admit this, but they know their real shortcomings as well as their merits, and the interest of the person himself in the thing to be criticised produces the subjective determination of the wit-work which would otherwise be difficult to bring about. Incidentally I do not know whether one often finds a people that makes merry so unreservedly over its own shortcomings.

As an illustration I can point to the story cited on page 112 in which the Jew in the train immediately abandons all sense of decency of deportment as soon as he recognizes the new arrival in his coupé as his coreligionist. We have come to know this joke as an illustration by means of a detail—representation through a trifle; it is supposed to represent the democratic mode of thought of the Jew who recognizes no difference between master and servant, but unfortunately this also disturbs discipline and co-operation. Another especially interesting series of jokes presents the relationship between the poor and the rich Jews: their heroes are the "shnorrer,"[1] and the charitable gentleman or the baron. *The shnorrer, who was a regular Sunday-dinner guest at a certain house, appeared one day accompanied by a young stranger, who prepared to seat himself at the table. "Who is that?" demanded the host. "He became my son-in-law last week," was the reply, "and I have agreed to supply his board for the first year."* The tendency of these stories is always the same, and is most distinctly shown in the following story. *The*

[1] An habitual beggar.

shnorrer supplicates the baron for money to visit the bathing resort Ostend, as the physician has ordered him to take sea-baths for his ailment. The baron remarks that Ostend is an especially expensive resort, and that a less fashionable place would do just as well. But the shnorrer rejects that proposition by saying, " Herr Baron, nothing is too expensive for my health." That is an excellent displacement-witticism which we could have taken as a model of its kind. The baron is evidently anxious to save his money, but the shnorrer replies as if the baron's money were his own, which he may then consider secondary to his health. One is forced to laugh at the insolence of the demand, but these jokes are exceptionally unequipped with a façade to becloud the understanding. The truth is that the shnorrer who mentally treats the rich man's money as his own, really possesses almost the right to this mistake, according to the sacred codes of the Jews. Naturally the resistance which is responsible for this joke is directed against the law which even the pious find very oppressing.

Another story relates *how on the steps of a rich man's house a shnorrer met one of his own kind. The latter counseled him to depart, saying, " Do not go up to-day, the Baron is out of sorts and refuses to give any one more than a dollar." " I will go up anyway," replied the first. " Why in the world should I make him a present of a dollar? Is he making me any presents? "*

This witticism makes use of the technique of absurdity by permitting the shnorrer to declare that the baron gives him nothing at the same moment in which he is preparing to beg him for the donation. But the absurdity is only apparent, for it is almost true that the rich man gives him nothing, since he is obligated by the mandate to give alms, and strictly speaking must be thankful that the shnorrer gives him an opportunity to be charitable. The ordinary, bourgeois conception of alms is at cross-purposes with the religious one; it openly revolts against the religious conception in the *story about the baron who, having been deeply touched by the shnorrer's tale of woe, rang for his servants and said: " Throw him out of the house; he is breaking my heart."* This obvious exposition of the tendency again creates a case of border-line wit. From the no longer witty complaint: " It is really no advantage to be a rich man among Jews. The foreign misery does not grant one the pleasure of one's own fortune," these last stories are distinguished only by the illustration of a single situation.

Other stories as the following, which, technically again presenting border-lines of wit, have their origin in a deeply pessimistic cynicism. *A patient whose hearing was defective consulted a physician who made the correct diagnosis, namely, that the patient probably drank too much whiskey and consequently was becoming deaf. He advised him to desist from drinking and the patient promised to follow his advice. Some time thereafter the doctor met him on the street and inquired in a loud voice about his condition. "Thank you, Doctor," was the reply, "there is no necessity for speaking so loudly, I have given up drinking whiskey and consequently I hear perfectly." Some time afterwards they met again. The doctor again inquired into his condition in the usual voice, but noticed that he did not make himself understood. "It seems to me that you are deaf again because you have returned to drinking whiskey," shouted the doctor in the patient's ear. "Perhaps you are right," answered the latter, "I have taken to drinking again, and I shall tell you why. As long as I did not drink I could hear, but all that I heard was not as good as the whiskey."* Technically this joke is nothing more than an illustration. The jargon and the ability of the *raconteur* must aid the producing of laughter.

But behind it there lies the sad question, "Is not the man right in his choice?"

It is the manifold hopeless misery of the Jews to which these pessimistical stories allude, which urged me to add them to tendency-wit.

Critical and Blasphemous Witticisms

Other jokes, cynical in a similar sense, and not only stories about Jews, attack religious dogmas and the belief in God Himself. The story about the "telepathic look of the rabbi," whose technique consisted in the faulty thinking which made phantasy equal to reality, (the conception of displacement is also tenable) is such a cynical or critical witticism directed against miracle-workers and also, surely, against belief in miracles. Heine is reported to have made a directly blasphemous joke as he lay dying. *When the kindly priest commended him to God's mercy and inspired him with the hope that God would forgive him his sins, he replied: " Bien sûr qu'il me pardonnera; c'est son métier."* That is a derogatory comparison; technically its value lies only in the allusion, for a métier—business or vocation —is plied either by a craftsman or a physician, and what is more he has only a single métier. The strength of the wit, however, lies in its téndency. The joke is intended to mean nothing else, but: Certainly he will forgive me; that is what he is here for, and for no other purpose have I engaged him (just as one retains one's doctor or one's lawyer). Thus, the helpless dying man is still conscious of the fact that he has created God for himself and has clothed Him with the power in order to make use of Him as occasion arises. The so-called creature makes itself known as the Creator only a short time before his extinction.

Skeptical Wit

To the three kinds of tendency-wit discussed so far—exhibitionistic or obscene wit, aggressive or hostile wit, and cynical wit (critical, blasphemous)—I desire to add a fourth and the most uncommon of all, whose character can be elucidated by a good example.

Two Jews met in a train at a Galician railway station. "Where are you traveling?" asked one. "To Cracow," was the reply. "Now see here, what a liar you are!" said the first one, bristling. "When you say that you are traveling to Cracow, you really wish me to believe that you are traveling to Lemberg. Well, but I am sure that you are really traveling to Cracow, so why lie about it?"

This precious story, which creates an impression of exaggerated subtlety, evidently operates by means of the technique of absurdity. The second Jew has put himself in the way of being called a liar because he has said that he is traveling to Cracow, which is his real goal! However, this strong technical means—absurdity—is paired here with another technique—representation through the opposite, for, according to the uncontradicted assertion of the first, the second one is lying when he speaks the truth, and speaks the truth by means of a lie. However, the more earnest content of this joke is the question of the conditions of truth; again the joke points to a problem and makes use of the uncertainty of one of our commonest notions. Does it constitute truth if one describes things as they are and does not concern himself with the way the hearers will interpret what one has said? Or is this merely Jesuitical truth, and does not the real truthfulness consist much more in having a regard for the hearer and of furnishing him an exact picture of his own mind? I consider jokes of this type sufficiently different from the others to assign them a special place. What they attack is not a person nor an institution, but the certainty of our very knowledge—one of our speculative gifts. Hence the name " skeptical " witticism will be the most expressive for them.

In the course of our discussion of the tendencies of wit we have gotten perhaps many an elucidation and certainly found numerous incentives for further investigations. But the results of this chapter combine with those of the preceding chapter to form a difficult problem. If it be true that the pleasure created by wit is dependent upon the technique on one hand and upon the tendency on the other hand, under what common point of view can these two utterly different pleasure-sources of wit be united?

B. SYNTHESIS

IV

WE can now definitely assert that we know from what sources the peculiar pleasure arises furnished us by wit. We know that we can be easily misled to mistake our sense of satisfaction experienced through the thought-content of the sentence for the actual pleasure derived from the wit, on the other hand, the latter itself has two intrinsic sources, namely, the wit-technique and the wit-tendency. What we now desire to ascertain is the manner in which pleasure originates from these sources and the mechanism of this resultant pleasure.

It seems to us that the desired explanation can be more easily ascertained in tendency-wit than in harmless wit. We shall therefore commence with the former.

The pleasure in tendency-wit results from the fact that a tendency, whose gratification would otherwise remain unfulfilled, is actually gratified. That such gratification is a source of pleasure is self-evident without further discussion. But the manner in which wit brings

about gratification is connected with special
conditions from which we may perhaps gain
further information. Here two cases must be
differentiated. The simpler case is the one in
which the gratification of the tendency is opposed by an external hindrance which is eluded
by the wit. This process we found, for example, in the reply which Serenissimus received
to his query whether the mother of the stranger
he addressed had ever sojourned in his home,
and likewise in the question of the art critic
who asked: "And where is the Savior?" when
the two rich rogues showed him their portraits.
In one case the tendency serves to answer one
insult with another; in the other case it offers
an affront instead of the demanded expert
opinion; in both cases the tendency was opposed by purely external factors, namely, the
powerful position of the persons who are the
targets of the insult. Nevertheless it may seem
strange to us that these and analogous tendency-witticisms have not the power to produce
a strong laughing effect, no matter how much
they may gratify us.

It is different, however, if no external factors but internal hindrances stand in the way
of the direct realization of the tendency, that
is, if an inner feeling opposes the tendency.
This condition, according to our assumption,

was present in the aggressive joke of Mr. N.
(p. 28) and in the one of Wendell Phillips, in
whom a strong inclination to use invectives was
stifled by a highly developed æsthetic sense.
With the aid of wit the inner resistances in
these special cases were overcome and the inhibition removed. As in the case of external
hindrances, the gratification of the tendency is
made possible, and a suppression with its concomitant " psychic damming " is thus obviated.
So far the mechanism of the development of
pleasure would seem to be identical in both
cases.

At this place, however, we are inclined to
feel that we should enter more deeply into the
differentiation of the psychological situation between the cases of external and internal hindrance, as we have a faint notion that the removal of the inner hindrance might possibly
result in a disproportionately higher contribution to pleasure. But I propose that we rest
content here, that we be satisfied for the present with this one collection of evidence which
adheres to what is essential to us. The only
difference between the cases of outer and inner
hindrances consists in the fact that here an already existing inhibition is removed, while
there the formation of a new inhibition is
avoided. We hardly resort to speculation when

we assert that a *" psychic expenditure "* is required for the formation as well as for the retention of a psychic inhibition. Now if we find that in both cases the use of the tendency-wit produces pleasure, then it may be assumed *that such resultant pleasure corresponds to the economy of psychic expenditure.*

Thus we are once more confronted with the principle of *economy* which we noticed first in the study of the technique of word-wit. But whereas the economy we believed to have found at first was in the use of few or possibly the same words, we can here foresee an economy of psychic expenditure in general in a far more comprehensive sense, and we think it possible to come nearer to the nature of wit through a better determination of the as yet very obscure idea of " psychic expenditure."

A certain amount of haziness which we could not dissipate during the study of the pleasure mechanism in tendency-wit we accept as a slight punishment for attempting to elucidate the more complicated problem before the simpler one, or the tendency-wit before the harmless wit. We observe that *" economy in the expenditure of inhibitions or suppressions "* seems to be the secret of the pleasurable effect of tendency-wit, and we now turn to the mechanism of the pleasure in harmless wit.

While examining appropriate examples of
harmless witticisms, in which we had no fear
of false judgment through content or tendency, we were forced to the conclusion that the
techniques of wit themselves are pleasure-
sources; now we wish to ascertain whether the
pleasure may be traced to the economy in
psychic expenditure. In a group of these witticisms (plays on words) the technique consisted in directing the psychic focus upon the
sound instead of upon the sense of the word,
and in allowing the (acoustic) word-disguise
to take the place of the meaning accorded to it
by its relations to reality. We are really justified in assuming that great relief is thereby afforded to the psychic work, and that in the
serious use of words we refrain from this convenient procedure only at the expense of a
certain amount of exertion, We can observe
that abnormal mental states, in which the possibility of concentrating psychic expenditure on
one place is probably restricted, actually allow
to come to the foreground word-sound associations of this kind rather than the significance of
the words, and that such patients react in their
speech with " outer " instead of " inner " associations. Also in children who are still accustomed to treat the word as an object we
notice the inclination to look for the same

meaning in words of the same or of similar sounds, which is a source of great amusement to adults. If we experience in wit an unmistakable pleasure because through the use of the same or similar words we reach from one set of ideas to a distant other one, (as in " Home-Roulard " from the kitchen to politics), we can justly refer this pleasure to the economy of psychic expenditure. The pleasure of the wit resulting from such a " short-circuit " appears greater the more remote and foreign the two series of ideas which become related through the same word are to each other, or the greater the economy in thought brought about by the technical means of wit. We may add that in this case wit makes use of a means of connection which is rejected by and carefully avoided in serious thinking.[1]

[1] If I may be permitted to anticipate what later is discussed in the text I can here throw some light upon the condition which seems to be authoritative in the usage of language when it is a question of calling a joke "good" or "poor." If by means of a double meaning or slightly modified word I have gotten from one idea to another by a short route, and if this does not also simultaneously result in senseful association between the two ideas, then I have made a "poor" joke. In this poor joke one word or the "point" forms the only existing association between the two widely separated ideas. The joke "Home-Roulard" used above is such an example. But a "good" joke results if the infantile expectation is right in the end and if with the similarity of the word another essential similarity in meaning is really simultaneously produced—as in the examples Traduttore—Traditore (translator—traitor), and Amantes—Amentes

A second group of technical means of wit—unification, similar sounding words, manifold application, modification of familiar idioms, allusions to quotations—all evince one common character, namely, that one always discovers something familiar where one expects to find something new instead. To discover the familiar is pleasurable and it is not difficult to recognize such pleasure as economy-pleasure and to refer it to the economy of psychic expenditure.

That the discovery of the familiar—"recognition"—causes pleasure seems to be universally admitted. Groos says:[1] "Recognition is everywhere bound up with feelings of pleas-

(lovers—lunatics). The two disparate ideas which are here linked by an outer association are held together besides by a senseful connection which expresses an important relationship between them. The outer association only replaces the inner connection; it serves to indicate the latter or to clarify it. Not only does "translator" sound somewhat similar to "traitor," but he is a sort of a traitor whose claims to that name are good. The same may be said of Amantes—Amentes. Not only do the words bear a resemblance, but the similarity between "love" and "lunacy" has been noted from time immemorial.

The distinction made here agrees with the differentiation, to be made later, between a "witticism" and a "jest." However, it would not be correct to exclude examples like Home-Roulard from the discussion of the nature of wit. As soon as we take into consideration the peculiar pleasure of wit, we discover that the "poor" witticisms are by no means poor as witticisms, i.e., they are by no means unsuited for the production of pleasure.

[1] *Die Spiele der Menschen*, 1899, p. 153.

ure where it has not been made too mechanica.
(as perhaps in dressing . . .). Even the mere
quality of acquaintanceship is easily accompanied by that gentle delight which Faust experiences when, after an uncanny experience, he
steps into his study." If the act of recognition
is so pleasureful, we may expect that man
merges into the habit of practicing this activity for its own sake, that is, he experiments
playfully with it. In fact, Aristotle recognized
in the joy of rediscovery the basis of artistic
pleasure, and it cannot be denied that this
principle must not be overlooked even if it has
not such a far-reaching significance as Aristotle assumes.

Groos then discusses the games, whose character consists of heightening the pleasure of
rediscovery by putting hindrances in its path,
or in other words by raising a " psychic dam "
which is removed by the act of recognition.
However, his attempted explanation leaves the
assumption that recognition as such is pleasurable, in that he attributes the pleasure of recognition connected with these games to the
pleasure in power or to the surmounting of a
difficulty. I consider this latter factor as secondary, and I find no occasion for abandoning
the simpler explanation, that the recognition
per se, i.e., through the alleviation of the psy-

chic expenditure, is pleasurable, and that the games founded upon this pleasure make use of the damming-mechanism merely in order to intensify their effect.

We know also that the source of pleasure in rhyme, alliteration, refrain, and other forms of repetition of similar sounding words in poetry, is due merely to the discovery of the familiar. A " sense of power " plays no perceptible rôle in these techniques, which show so marked an agreement with the " manifold application " in wit.

Considering the close connection between recognition and remembering, the assumption is no longer daring that there exists also a pleasure in remembering, i.e., that the act of remembering in itself is accompanied by a feeling of pleasure of a similar origin. Groos seems to have no objection to such an assumption, but he again deducts the pleasure of remembering from the " sense of power " in which he seeks— as I believe unjustly—the principal basis of pleasure in almost all games.

The Factor of Actuality

The use of another technical expedient of wit, which has not yet been mentioned, is also dependent upon " the rediscovery of the fa-

miliar." I refer to the factor of *actuality*
(dealing with actual persons, things, or events),
which in many witticisms provides a prolific
source of pleasure and explains several peculiarities in the life history of wit. There are
witticisms which are entirely free from this condition, and in a treatise on wit it is incumbent
upon us to make use of such examples almost
exclusively. But we must not forget that we
laughed perhaps more heartily over such peren-
nial witticisms than over others; witticisms
whose application now would be difficult, because they would require long commentaries,
and even with that aid the former effect could
not be attained. These latter witticisms contained allusions to persons and occurrences
which were " actual " at the time, which had
stimulated general interest and were endowed
with tension. After the cessation of this
interest, after the settlement of these particular affairs, the witticisms lost a part of
their pleasurable effect, and a very considerable. Thus, for example, the joke which
my friendly host made when he called
the dish that was being served a " Home-
Roulard," seems to me by no means as good
now as when the question of Home Rule was
a continuous headline in the political columns
of our newspaper. If I now attempt to ex-

press my appreciation of this joke by stating
that this one word led us from the idea of the
kitchen to the distant field of politics, and
saved us a long mental detour, I should have
been forced at that time to change this description as follows: " That this word led us from
the idea of the kitchen to the very distant field
of politics; but that our lively interest was all
the keener because this question was constantly
absorbing us." The same thing is true of
another joke: *" This girl reminds me of
Dreyfus; the army does not believe in her innocence,"* which has become blurred in spite of
the fact that its technical means has remained
unchanged. The confusion arising from the
comparison with, and the double meaning of,
the word " innocence " cannot do away with the
fact that the allusion, which at that time
touched upon a matter pregnant with excitement, now recalls an interest set at rest. The
many irresistible jokes about the present war
will sink in our estimation in a very short time.

A great many witticisms in circulation reach
a certain age or rather go through a course
composed of a flourishing season and a mature
season, and then sink into complete oblivion.
The need that people feel to draw pleasure
from their mental processes continually creates
new witticisms which are supported by current

interests of the day. The vitality of actual witticisms is not their own, it is borrowed by way
of allusion from those other interests, the ex-
piration of which determines the fate of the
witticism. The factor of actuality which may
be added as a transitory pleasure-source of wit,
although it is productive in itself, cannot be
simply put on the same basis as the rediscovery
of the familiar. It is much more a question of
a special qualification of the familiar which
must be aided by the quality of freshness and
recency and which has not been affected by for-
getfulness. In the formation of the dream one
also finds that there is a special preference for
what is recent, and one cannot refrain from in-
ferring that the association with what is recent
is rewarded or facilitated by a special pleasure premium.

Unification, which is really nothing more
than repetition in the sphere of mental association instead of in material, has been accorded an especial recognition as a pleasure-
source of wit by G. Th. Fechner.[1] He says:
"In my opinion the principle of uniform connection of the manifold, plays the most important rôle in the field under discussion; it
needs, however, the support of subsidiary determinations in order to drive across the thresh-

[1] *Vorschule der Aesthetik*, 1, XVII.

old the pleasure with its peculiar character which the cases here belonging can furnish." [1]

In all of these cases of repetition of the same association or of the same word-material, of re-finding the familiar and recent, we surely cannot be prevented from referring the pleasure thereby experienced to the economy in psychic expenditure; providing that this viewpoint proves fertile for the explanation of single facts as well as for bringing to light new generalities. We are fully conscious of the fact that we have yet to make clear the manner in which this economy results and also the meaning of the expression " psychic expenditure."

The third group of the technique of wit, mostly thought-wit, which includes false logic, displacement, absurdity, representation through the opposite, and other varieties, may seem at first sight to present special features and to be unrelated to the techniques of the discovery of the familiar, or the replacing of object-associations by word-associations. But it will not be difficult to demonstrate that this group, too, shows an economy or facilitation of psychic expenditure.

It is quite obvious that it is easier and more convenient to turn away from a definite trend of thought than to stick to it; it is easier to

[1] Chapter XVII.

mix up different things than to distinguish
them; and it is particularly easier to travel
over modes of reasoning unsanctioned by logic;
finally in connecting words or thoughts it is
especially easy to overlook the fact that such
connections should result in sense. All this is
indubitable and this is exactly what is done by
the techniques of the wit in question. It will
sound strange, however, to assert that such
processes in the wit-work may produce pleasure, since outside of wit we can experience only
unpleasant feelings of defense against all these
kinds of inferior achievement of our mental activity.

Word-pleasure and Pleasure in Nonsense

The " pleasure in nonsense," as we may call
it for short, is, in the seriousness of our life,
crowded back almost to the vanishing point.
To demonstrate it we must enter into the study
of two cases in one of which it is still visible
and in the other becomes visible for the second
time. I refer to the behavior of the learning
child and to the behavior of the adult under un-
stable toxic influences. When the child learns
to control the vocabulary of its mother tongue
it apparently takes great pleasure in " ex-
perimenting playfully " with that material

(Groos) ; it connects words without regard for their meaning in order to obtain pleasure from the rhyme and rhythm. Gradually the child is deprived of this pleasure until only the sense-ful connection of words is allowed him. But even in later life there is still a tendency to overstep the acquired restrictions in the use of words, a tendency which manifests itself in disfiguring the same by definite appendages, and in changing their forms by means of certain contrivances (reduplication, trembling speech) or even by developing an individual language for use in playing,—efforts which re-appear also among the insane of a certain category.

I believe that whatever the motive which actuated the child when it began such playings, in its further development the child indulges in them fully conscious that they are nonsensical and derives pleasure from this stimulus which is interdicted by reason. It now makes use of play in order to withdraw from the pressure of critical reason. More powerful, however, are the restrictions which must develop in education along the lines of right thinking and in the separation of reality from fiction, and it is for this reason that the resistance against the pressures of thinking and reality is far-reaching and persistent; even the phenomena of phantasy formation come under this point of view. The power of reason usually grows so strong during the later part of childhood and during that period of education which extends over the age of puberty, that the pleasure in " freed nonsense " rarely dares manifest itself. One fears to utter nonsense; but it seems to me that the inclination characteristic of boys to act in a contradictory and inexpedient manner is a direct outcome of this pleasure in nonsense. In pathological cases one often sees this tendency so accentuated that it again controls the speeches and answers of the pupils. In the case of some college students who merged into neuroses I could convince myself that the unconscious pleasure derived from the nonsense produced by them is just as much responsible for their mistakes as their actual ignorance.

Reproduction of Old Liberties

The student does not give up his demonstrations against the pressures of thinking and reality whose domination becomes unceasingly intolerant and unrestricted. A good part of the tendency of students to skylarking is responsible for this reaction. Man is an " untiring pleasure seeker "—I can no longer recall

which author coined this happy expression—
and finds it extremely difficult to renounce
pleasure once experienced. With the hilarious
nonsense of "sprees" (*Bierschwefel*), college
cries, and songs, the student attempts to pre-
serve that pleasure which results from freedom
of thought, a freedom of which he is more and
more deprived through scholastic discipline.
Even much later, when as a mature man he
meets with others at scientific congresses and
class reunions and feels himself a student
again, he must read at the end of the session
the "*Kneipzeitung*," or the comic college paper,
which distorts the newly gained knowledge into
the nonsensical and thus compensates him for the
newly added mental inhibitions.

The very terms "*Bierschwefel*" and "*Kneipzeitung*" are proof that the reason which has
stifled the pleasure in nonsense has become so
powerful that not even temporarily can it be
abandoned without toxic agency. The change
in the state of mind is the most valuable thing
that alcohol offers man, and that is the reason
why this "poison" is not equally indispensable
for all people. The hilarious humor, whether
due to endogenous origin or whether produced
toxically, weakens the inhibiting forces among
which is reason and thus again makes accessible pleasure-sources which are burdened by

suppression. It is very instructive to see how the demand made upon wit sinks with the rise in spirits. The latter actually replace wit, just as wit must make an effort to replace the mental state in which the otherwise inhibited pleasure possibilities (pleasure in nonsense among the rest) assert themselves.

"With little wit and much comfort."

Under the influence of alcohol the adult again becomes a child who derives pleasure from the free disposal of his mental stream without being restricted by the pressure of logic.

We hope we have shown that the technique of absurdity in wit corresponds to a source of pleasure. We need hardly repeat that this pleasure results from the economy of psychic expenditure or alleviation from the pressure of reason.

On reviewing again the wit-technique classified under three headings we notice that the first and last of these groups—the replacement of object-association by word-association, and the use of absurdity as a restorer of old liberties and as a relief from the pressure of intellectual upbringing—can be taken collectively. Psychic relief may in a way be compared to economy, which constitutes the technique of the second group. Alleviation of the already existing psychic expenditure, and economy in the yet to be offered psychic expenditure, are two principles from which all techniques of wit and with them all pleasure in these techniques can be deduced. The two forms of the technique and the resultant pleasures correspond more or less in general to the division of wit into word- and thought-witticisms.

Play and Jest

The preceding discussions have led us unexpectedly to an understanding of the history of the development of psychogenesis of wit which we shall now examine still further. We have become acquainted with the successive steps in wit, the development of which up to tendency-wit will undoubtedly reveal new relationships between the different characters of wit. Antedating wit there exists something which we may designate as " play " or " jest." Play—we shall retain this name—appears in children while they are learning how to use words and connect thoughts; this playing is probably the result of an impulse which urges the child to exercise its capacities (Groos). During this process it experiences pleasurable effects which originate from the repetition of similarities, the rediscovery of the familiar, sound-associations, etc., which may be explained as an unexpected economy of psychic expenditure. Therefore it surprises no one that these resulting pleasures urge the child to practice playing and impel it to continue without regard for the meaning of words or the connections between sentences. Playing with words and thoughts, motivated by certain pleasures in economy, would thus be the first step of wit.

This playing is stopped by the growing strength of a factor which may well be called criticism or reason. The play is then rejected as senseless or as directly absurd, and by virtue of reason it becomes impossible. Only accidentally is it now possible to derive pleasure from those sources of rediscovery of the familiar, etc., which is explained by the fact that the maturing person has then merged into a playful mood which, as in the case of merriment in the child, removes inhibitions. In this way only is the old pleasure-giving playing made possible, but as men do not wish to wait for these propitious occasions and also hate to forego this pleasure, they seek means to make themselves independent of these pleasant states. The further development of wit is directed by these two impulses; the one striving to elude reason and the other to substitute for the adult an infantile state of mind.

This gives rise to the second stage of wit, the *jest* (*Scherz*). The object of the jest is to bring about the resultant pleasure of playing and at the same time appease the protesting reason which strives to suppress the pleasant feeling. There is but one way to accomplish this. The senseless combination of words or the absurd linking of thoughts must make sense after all. The whole process of wit production is therefore directed towards the discovery of words and thought constellations which fulfill these conditions. The jest makes use of almost all the technical means of wit, and usage of language makes no consequential distinction between jest (*Scherz*) and wit (*Witz*). What distinguishes the jest from wit is the fact that the pith of the sentence withdrawn from criticism does not need to be valuable, new, or even good; it matters only that it can be expressed, even though what it may say is obsolete, superfluous, and useless. The most conspicuous factor of the jest is the gratification it affords by making possible that which reason forbids.

A mere jest is the following of Professor Kästner, who taught physics at Göttingen in the 16th century, and who was fond of making jokes. Wishing to enroll a student named Warr in his class, he asked him his age, and upon receiving the reply that he was thirty years of age he exclaimed: "Aha, so I have the honor of seeing the thirty years' War."[1] When asked what vocations his sons followed Rokitansky jestingly answered: "Two are healing and two are howling," (two physicians and two singers). The reply was correct and therefore unimpeachable, but it added nothing to what is contained in the parenthetic expression. There is no doubt that the answer assumed another form only because of the pleasure which arises from the unification and assonance of both words.

I believe that we now see our way clear. In estimating the techniques of wit we were constantly disturbed by the fact that these are not peculiar to wit alone, and yet the nature of wit seemed to depend upon them, since their removal by means of reduction nullified the character as well as the pleasure of wit. Now we become aware that what we have described as techniques of wit—and which in a certain sense we shall have to continue to call so—are really the sources from which wit derives pleasure; nor does it strike us as strange that other processes draw from the same sources with the same object in view. The technique, however, which is peculiar to and belongs to wit alone consists in a process of safeguarding the use

[1] Kleinpaul: *Die Rätsel der Sprache*, 1890.

of this pleasure-forming means against the protest of reason which would obviate the pleasure. We can make few generalizations about this process. The wit-work, as we have already remarked, expresses itself in the selection of such word-material and such thought-situations as to permit the old play with words and thoughts to stand the test of reason; but to accomplish this end the cleverest use must be made of all the peculiarities of the stock of words and of all constellations of mental combinations. Later on perhaps we shall be in a position to characterize the wit-work by a definite attribute; for the present it must remain unexplained how our wit makes its advantageous selections. The tendency and capacity of wit to guard the pleasure-forming word and thought combinations against reason, already makes itself visible as an essential criterion in jests. From the beginning its object is to remove inner inhibitions and thereby render productive those pleasure-sources which have become inaccessible, and we shall find that it remains true to this characteristic throughout the course of its entire development.

We are now in a position to prescribe a correct place for the factor " sense in nonsense," (see Introduction, page 8), to which the authors ascribe so much significance in respect to the

recognition of wit and the explanation of the
pleasurable effect. The two firmly established
points in the determination of wit—its tendency
to carry through the pleasureful play, and its
effort to guard it against the criticism of reason
—make it perfectly clear why the individual
witticism, even though it appear nonsensical
from one point of view, must appear full of
meaning or at least acceptable from another.
How it accomplishes this is the business of the
wit-work; if it is not successful it is relegated
to the category of "nonsense." Nor do we find
it necessary to deduce the resultant pleasure
of wit from the conflict of feelings which
emerge either directly or by way of "confusion and clearness," from the simultaneous
sense and nonsense of the wit. There is just
as little necessity for our delving deeper into
the question how pleasure can come from the
succession of that part of the wit considered
senseless and from that part recognized as
senseful. The psychogenesis of wit has taught
us that the pleasure of wit arises from word-
play or from the liberation of nonsense, and
that the sense of wit is meant only to
guard this pleasure against suppression through
reason.

Jest and Wit

Thus the problem of the essential character of wit could almost be explained by means of the jest. We may follow the development of the jest until it reaches its height in the tendency-wit. The jest gives tendency a prior position when it is a question of supplying us with pleasure, and it is content when its utterance does not appear utterly senseless or insipid. But if this utterance is substantial and valuable the jest changes into wit. A thought, which would have been worthy of our interest even when expressed in the most unpretentious form, is now invested in a form which must in itself excite our sense of satisfaction. Such an association we cannot help thinking certainly has not come into existence unintentionally; we must make effort to divine the intention at the bottom of the formation of wit. An incidental observation, made once before, will put us on the right track. We have already remarked that a good witticism gives us, so to speak, a general feeling of satisfaction without our being able to decide offhand which part of the pleasure comes from the witty form and which part from the excellent thought contained in the context (p. 131). We are deceiving ourselves constantly about this division; sometimes we overvalue the quality of the wit on account of our admiration for the thought contained therein, and then again we overestimate the value of the thought on account of the pleasure afforded us by the witty investment. We know not what gives us pleasure nor at what we are laughing. This uncertainty of our judgment, assuming it to be a fact, may have given the motive for the formation of wit in the literal sense. The thought seeks the witty disguise because it thereby recommends itself to our attention and can thus appear to us more important and valuable than it really is; but above all because this disguise fascinates and confuses our reason. We are apt to attribute to the thought the pleasure derived from the witty form, and we are not inclined to consider improper what has given us pleasure, and in this way deprive ourselves of a source of pleasure. For if wit made us laugh it was because it established in us a mood most unfavorable to reason, which in turn has forced upon us that state of mind which was once contented with mere playing and which wit has attempted to replace with all the means at its command. Although we have already established the fact that such wit is harmless and does not yet show a tendency, we may not deny that, strictly speaking, it is the jest alone which shows no tendency; that is, it serves to produce pleasure only. For wit is really never purposeless even if the thought contained therein shows no tendency and merely serves a theoretical, intellectual interest. Wit carries out its purpose in advancing the thought by magnifying it and by guarding it against reason. Here again it reveals its original nature in that it sets itself up against an inhibiting and restrictive power, or against the critical judgment.

The first use of wit, which goes beyond the mere production of pleasure, points out the road to be followed. Wit is now recognized as a powerful psychic factor whose weight can decide the issue if it falls into this or that side of the scale. The great tendencies and impulses of our psychic life enlist its service for their own purposes. The original purposeless wit, which began as play, becomes related in a *secondary* manner to tendencies from which nothing that is formed in psychic life can escape for any length of time. We already know what it can achieve in the service of the exhibitionistic, aggressive, cynical, and sceptical tendencies. In the case of obscene wit, which originated in the smutty joke, it makes a confederate of the third person who originally disturbed the sexual situation, by giving him pleasure through the utterance which causes the woman to be ashamed in his presence. In the case of the aggressive tendency, wit by the same means changes the original indifferent hearers into active haters and scorners, and in this way confronts the enemy with a host of opponents where formerly there was but one. In the first case it overcomes the inhibitions of shame and decorum by the pleasure premium which it offers. In the second case it overthrows the critical judgment which would otherwise have examined the dispute in question. In the third and fourth cases where wit is in the service of the cynical and sceptical tendency, it shatters the respect for institutions and truths in which the hearer had believed, first by strengthening the argument, and secondly by resorting to a new method of attack. Where the argument seeks to draw the hearer's reason to its side, wit strives to push aside this reason. There is no doubt that wit has chosen the way which is psychologically more efficacious.

The Development into Tendency-wit

What impressed us in reviewing the achievements of tendency-wit was the effect it produced on the hearer. It is more important, however, to understand the effect produced by wit on the psychic life of the person who makes it, or more precisely expressed, on the psychic life of the person who conceives it. Once before we have expressed the intention, which we find occasion to repeat here, that we wish to study the psychic processes of wit in regard to its apportionment between two persons. We can assume for the present that the psychic process aroused by wit in the hearer is usually an imitation of the psychic processes of the wit producer. The outer inhibitions which are to be overcome in the hearer correspond to the inner inhibitions of the wit producer. In the latter the expectation of the outer hindrance exists, at least as an inhibiting idea. The inner hindrance, which is overcome in tendency-wit, is evident in some single cases; for example, in Mr. N.'s joke (p. 28) we can assume that it not only enables the hearer to enjoy the pleasure of the aggression through injuries but it also makes it possible for him to produce the wit in the first place. Of the different kinds of inner inhibitions or suppressions one is especially worthy of our interest because it is the most far-reaching. We designate that form by the term " repression." It is characterized by the fact that it excludes from consciousness certain former emotions and their products. We shall learn that tendency-wit itself is capable of liberating pleasure from sources that have undergone repression. If the overcoming of outer hindrances can be referred, in the manner indicated above, to inner inhibitions and repressions we may say that tendency-wit proves more clearly than any other developmental stage of wit that the main character of wit-making is to set free pleasure by removing inhibitions. It reinforces tendencies to which it gives its services by bringing them assistance from repressed emotions; or it puts itself at the disposal of the repressed tendencies directly.

One may readily concede that these are the functions of tendency-wit, but one must nevertheless admit that we do not understand in what manner these functions can succeed in accomplishing their end. The power of tendency-wit consists in the pleasure which it derives from the sources of word-plays and liberated nonsense, and if one can judge from the impressions received from purposeless jests, one cannot possibly consider the amount of the pleasure so great as to believe that it has the power to annul deep-rooted inhibitions and repressions. As a matter of fact we do not deal here with a simple propelling power but rather with a more complicated mechanism. Instead of covering the long circuitous route through which I arrived at an understanding of this re- lationship, I shall endeavor to demonstrate it by a short synthetic route.

G. Th. Fechner has established the principle of æsthetic assistance or enhancement which he explains in the following words: *"From the unopposed meeting of pleasurable states (Be- dingungen) which individually accomplish lit- tle, there results a greater, often much greater resultant pleasure than is warranted by the sum of the pleasure values of the separate states, or a greater result than could be ac- counted for as the sum of the individual ef- fects; in fact the mere meeting of this kind can result in a positive pleasure product which overflows the threshold of pleasure when the factors taken separately are too weak to ac- complish this. The only condition is that in comparison to others they must produce a greater sense of satisfaction."* [1] I am of the opinion that the theme of wit does not give us the opportunity to test the correctness of this principle which is demonstrable in many other artistic fields. But from wit we have learned something, which at least comes near this prin- ple, namely, that in a co-operation of many

[1] *Vorschule der Aesthetik*, Vol. 1, V, p. 51, 2nd Ed., Leipzig, 1897.

pleasure-producing factors we are in no position to assign to each one the resultant part which really belongs to it (see p. 131). But the situation assumed in the principle of assistance can be varied, and for these new conditions we can formulate the following combination of questions which are worthy of a reply. What usually happens if in one constellation there is a meeting of pleasurable and painful conditions? Upon what depends the result and the previous intimations of the result? Tendency-wit particularly shows these possibilities. There is one feeling or impulse which strives to liberate pleasure from a certain source and under unrestricted conditions certainly would liberate it, but there is another impulse which works against this development of pleasure, that is, which inhibits or suppresses it. The suppressing stream, as the result shows, must be somewhat stronger than the one suppressed, which however is by no means destroyed.

The Fore-pleasure Principle

But now there appears another impulse which strives to set free pleasure by this identical process, even though from different sources it thus acts like the suppressed stream. What can be the result in such a case? An example can make this clearer than this schematization.

There is an impulse to insult a certain person; but this is so strongly opposed by a feeling of decorum and æsthetic culture that the impulse to insult must be crushed. If, for example, by virtue of some changed emotional state the insult should happen to break through, this insulting tendency would subsequently be painfully perceived. Therefore the insult is omitted. There is a possibility, however, of making good wit from the words or thoughts which would have served in the insult; that is, pleasure can be set free from other sources without being hindered by the same suppression. But the second development of pleasure would have to be foregone if the insulting quality of the wit were not allowed to come out, and as the latter is allowed to come to the surface, it is connected with the new release of pleasure. Experience with tendency-wit shows that under such circumstances the suppressed tendency can become so strengthened by the aid of wit-pleasure as to overcome the otherwise stronger inhibition. One resorts to insults because wit is thereby made impossible. But the satisfaction thus obtained is not produced by wit alone; it is incomparably greater, in fact it is by so much greater than the pleasure of the wit, that we must assume that the former suppressed tendency has succeeded in breaking

through, perhaps without the need of an out-
let. Under these circumstances tendency-wit
causes the most prolific laughter.

Perhaps the investigation of the determinations of laughter will aid us in forming a
clearer picture of the process of the aid of wit
against suppression. But we see even now
that the case of tendency-wit is a special case
of the principle of aid. A possibility of the
development of pleasure enters into a situation
in which another pleasure possibility is so
hindered that individually it would not result
in pleasure. The result is a development of
pleasure which is greater by far than the added
possibility. The latter acted, as it were, as an
alluring premium; with the aid of a small sum
of pleasure a very large and almost inaccessible amount is obtained. I have good grounds
for thinking that this principle corresponds to
an arrangement which holds true in many
widely separated spheres of the psychic life,
and I consider it appropriate to designate the
pleasure serving to liberate the large sum of
pleasure as *fore-pleasure* and the principle as
the *principle* of *fore-pleasure.*

Play-pleasure and Removal-pleasure

The effect of tendency-wit may now be
formulated as follows: It enters the service of

tendencies in order to produce new pleasure by removing suppressions and repressions. This it does, using wit-pleasure as fore-pleasure. When we now review its development we may say that wit has remained true to its nature from beginning to end. It begins as play in order to obtain pleasure from the free use of words and thoughts. As soon as the growing reason forbids this senseless play with words and thoughts, it turns to the jest or joke in order to hold to these sources of pleasure and in order to be able to gain new pleasure from the liberation of the absurd. In the rôle of harmless wit it assists the thoughts and fortifies them against the impugnment of the critical judgment, whereby it makes use of the principle of intermingling the pleasure-sources. Finally, it enters into the great struggling suppressed tendencies in order to remove inner inhibitions in accordance with the principle of fore-pleasure. Reason, critical judgment, and suppression, these are the forces which it combats in turn. It firmly holds on to the original word-pleasure sources, and beginning with the stage of the jest opens for itself new pleasure sources by removing inhibition. The pleasure which it produces, be it play-pleasure or removal-pleasure, can at all times be traced to the economy of psychic expenditure, in so far as such a conception does not contradict the nature of pleasure, and proves itself productive also in other fields.[1]

[1] The nonsense-witticisms, which have been somewhat slighted in this treatise, deserve a short supplementary comment.

In view of the significance attributed by our conception to the factor "sense in nonsense," one might be tempted to demand that every witticism should be a nonsense-joke. But this is not necessary, because only the play with thoughts inevitably leads to nonsense, whereas the other source of wit-pleasure, the play with words, makes this impression incidental and does not regularly invoke the criticism connected with it. The double root of wit-pleasure—from the play with words and thoughts, which corresponds to the most important division into word- and thought-witticisms—sets its face against a short formulation of general principles about wit as a tangible aggravation of difficulties. The play with words produces laughter, as is well known, in consequence of the factor of recognition described above, and therefore suffers suppression only in a small degree. The play with thoughts cannot be motivated through such pleasure: it has suffered a very energetic suppression and the pleasure which it can give is only the pleasure of released inhibitions. Accordingly one may say that wit-pleasure shows a kernel of the original play-pleasure and a shell of removal-pleasure. Naturally we do not grant that the pleasure in nonsense-wit is due to the fact that we have succeeded in making nonsense despite the suppression, while we do notice that the play with words gives us pleasure. Nonsense, which has remained fixed in thought wit, acquires secondarily the function of stimulating our attention through confusion, it serves as a reinforcement of the effect of wit, but only when it is insistent, so that the confusion can anticipate the intellect by a definite fraction of time. That nonsense in wit may also be employed to represent a judgment contained within the thought has been demonstrated by the example on p. 73. But even this is not the primal signification of nonsense in wit.

A series of wit-like productions for which we have no appropriate name, but which may lay claim to the designation of "witty nonsense," may be added to the nonsense-jokes. They are very numerous, but I shall cite only two examples: As the fish was served to a guest at the table he put both hands twice into the mayonnaise and then ran them through his hair. Being looked at by his neighbor with astonishment he seemed to have noticed his mistake and excused himself, saying: "Pardon me, I thought it was spinach."

Or: "Life is like a suspension bridge," said the one. "How is that?" asked the other. "How should I know?" was the answer.

These extreme examples produce an effect through the fact that they give rise to the expectation of wit, so that one makes the effort to find the hidden sense behind the nonsense. But none is found, they are really nonsense. Under that deception it was possible for one moment to liberate the pleasure in nonsense. These witticisms are not altogether without tendencies, they furnish the narrator a certain pleasure in that they deceive and annoy the hearer. The latter then calms his anger by resolving that he himself should take the place of the narrator.

V

THE MOTIVES OF WIT AND WIT AS A SOCIAL PROCESS

IT seems superfluous to speak of the motives of wit, since the purpose of obtaining pleasure must be recognized as a sufficient motive of the wit-work. But on the one hand it is not impossible that still other motives participate in the production of wit, and on the other hand, in view of certain well-known experiences, the theme of the subjective determination of wit must be discussed.

Two things above all urge us to it. Though wit-making is an excellent means of obtaining pleasure from the psychic processes, we know that not all persons are equally able to make use of it. Wit-making is not at the disposal of all, in general there are but a few persons to whom one can point and say that they are witty. Here wit seems to be a special ability somewhere within the region of the old "psychic faculties," and this shows itself in its appearance as fairly independent of the other faculties such as intelligence, phantasy, memory, etc. A special talent or psychic de-

termination permitting or favoring wit-making
must be presupposed in all wit-makers.

I am afraid that we shall not get very far
in the exploration of this theme. Only now
and then do we succeed in proceeding from
the understanding of a single witticism to the
knowledge of the subjective determinations in
the mind of the wit-maker. It is quite accidental that the example of wit with which we
began our investigation of the wit-technique
permits us also to gain some insight into the
subjective determination of the witticism. I
am referring to Heine's witticism, to which also
Heymans and Lipps have paid attention.

"*I was sitting next to Solomon Rothschild
and he treated me just as an equal, quite famillionaire*" ("Bäder von Lucca").

Subjective Determination of the "Famillion-
aire" Witticism

Heine put this word in the mouth of a comical person, Hirsch-Hyacinth, collector, oper-
ator and tax appraiser from Hamburg, and
valet of the aristocratic baron, Cristoforo Gum-
pelino (formerly Gumpel). Evidently the
poet has experienced great pleasure in these
productions, for he allows Hirsch-Hyacinth to
talk big and puts in his mouth the most amus-

ing and most candid utterances; he positively endows him with the practical wisdom of a Sancho Panza. It is a pity that Heine, as it seems, had no liking for this dramatic figure and that he drops the delightful character so soon. From many passages it would seem that the poet himself is speaking behind the transparent mask of Hirsch-Hyacinth, and we are quite convinced that this person is nothing but a parody of the poet himself. Hirsch tells of reasons why he has discarded his former name and now calls himself Hyacinth. "Besides I have the advantage," he continues, "of having an H on my seal already, and therefore I am in no need of having a new letter engraved." But Heine himself resorted to this economy when he changed his surname "Harry" to "Heinrich" at his baptism. Every one acquainted with the life of the poet will recall that in Hamburg, where one also meets the personage Hirsch-Hyacinth, Heine had an uncle of the same name, who played the greatest rôle in Heine's life as the wealthy member of the family. The uncle's name was likewise Solomon, just like the elderly Rothschild who treated the impecunious Hirsch on such a famillionaire basis. What seems to be merely a jest in the mouth of Hirsch-Hyacinth soon reveals a background of earnest bitterness when we attribute it to the nephew Harry-Heinrich. For he belonged to the family, nay, more, it was his earnest wish to marry a daughter of this uncle, but she refused him, and his uncle always treated him on a somewhat famillionaire basis, as a poor relative. His rich relatives in Hamburg always dealt with him condescendingly. I recall the story of one of his old aunts by marriage who, when she was still young and pretty, sat next to some one at a family dinner who seemed to her unprepossessing and whom the other members of the family treated shabbily. She did not feel herself called upon to be any more condescending towards him. Only many years later did she discover that the careless and neglected cousin was the poet Heinrich Heine. We know from many a record how keenly Heine suffered from these repulses at the hands of his wealthy relatives in his youth and during later years. The witticism "famillionaire" grew out of the soil of such a subjective emotional feeling.

One may suspect similar subjective determinations in many other witticisms of the great scoffers, but I know of no other example by which one can show this in such a convincing way. It is therefore hazardous to venture a more definite opinion about the nature of this personal determination. Furthermore, one is not inclined in the first place to claim similar complicated conditions for the origin of each and every witticism. Neither are the witty productions of other celebrated men better suited to give us the desired insight into the subjective determination of wit. In fact, one gets the impression that the subjective determination of wit production is oftentimes not unrelated to persons suffering from neurotic diseases, when, for example, one learns that Lichtenberg was a confirmed hypochondriac burdened with all kinds of eccentricities. The great majority of witticisms, especially those produced from current happenings, are anonymous; one might be inquisitive to know what kind of people they are who originate them. The physician occasionally has an opportunity to make a study of persons who, if not renowned wits, are recognized in their circle as witty and as originators of many passable witticisms; he is often surprised to find such persons showing dissociated personalities and a predisposition to nervous affections. However, owing to insufficient data, we certainly cannot maintain that such a psychoneurotic constitution is a regular or necessary subjective condition for wit-making.

A clearer case is afforded by Jewish witticisms which, as before mentioned, are made exclusively by Jews themselves, whereas Jewish stories of different origin rarely rise above the level of the comical strain or of brutal mockery (p. 166). The determination for the self-participation here, as in Heine's joke "famillionaire," seems to be due to the fact that the person finds it difficult to express directly his criticism or aggression and is thus compelled to resort to by-ways.

Other subjective determinations or favorable conditions for wit-making are less shrouded in darkness. The motive for the production of harmless wit is usually the ambitious impulse to display one's spirit or to "show off." It is an impulse comparable to the impulse toward sexual exhibition. The existence of numerous inhibited impulses whose suppression retains some weakness produces a state favorable for the production of tendency-wit. Thus certain single components of the sexual constitution may appear as motives for wit-formation. A whole series of obscene witticisms lead one to the conclusion that a person who gives origin to such wit conceals a desire to exhibit. Persons having a powerful sadistical component in their sexuality, which is more or less inhibited in life, are most successful with the tendency-wit of aggression.

The Impulse to Impart Wit

The second fact which impels one to examine the subjective determination of wit is the common experience that nobody is satisfied with making wit for himself. Wit-making is inseparably connected with the desire to impart it; in fact this impulse is so strong that it is often realized after overcoming strong objections. In the comic, too, one experiences pleasure by imparting it to another person; but this is not imperative; one can enjoy the comic alone when one happens on it. Wit, on the other hand, must be imparted. Apparently the process of wit-formation does not end with the conception of wit. There remains something which strives to complete the mysterious process of wit-formation by imparting it.

We cannot conjecture, in the first place, what may have motivated the impulse to impart wit. But in wit we notice another peculiarity which again distinguishes it from the comic. If I encounter the latter I can laugh heartily over it alone; I am naturally pleased if by imparting it to some one else I make him laugh too. In the case of wit, however, which occurs to me or which I have made, I cannot laugh over it in spite of the unmistakable feeling of pleasure which I experience in the wit-

ticism. It is possible that my need to impart
the witticism to another is in some way connected with the resultant laughter, which is
manifest in the other, but denied to me.

But why do I not laugh over my own joke?
And what rôle does the other person play in
it?

Let us consider the last query first. In the
comic usually two persons come into consideration. Besides my own ego here is another person in whom I find something comic; if objects appear comical to me, it takes place by
means of a sort of personification which is not
uncommon in our notional life. The comic
process is satisfied with these two persons, the
ego and the object person; there may also be
a third person, but it is not obligatory Wit
as a play with one's own words and thoughts
at first dispenses with an object person, but
already, upon the first step of the jest, it demands another person to whom it can impart
its result, if it has succeeded in safeguarding
play and nonsense against the remonstrance
of reason. The second person in wit does not,
however, correspond to the object person, but
to the third person who is the other person in
the comic. It seems that in the jest the decision as to whether wit has fulfilled its task is
transferred to the other person, as if the ego

were not quite certain of its opinion in the matter. The harmless wit is also in need of the other person's support in order to ascertain whether it has accomplished its purpose. If wit enters the service of sexual or hostile tendencies, it can be described as a psychic process among three persons, just as in the comic, with the exception that there the third person plays a different rôle. The psychic process of wit is consummated here between the first person—the ego, and the third person —the stranger, and not, as in the comic, between the ego and the object person.

Also, in the case of the third person of wit, the wit is confronted with subjective determinations which can make the goal of the pleasure-stimulus unattainable. As Shakespeare says in *Love's Labor's Lost* (Act V, Scene 2):

> " A jest's prosperity lies in the ear
>   Of him that hears it, never in the tongue
>   Of him that makes it."

He whose thoughts run in sober channels is incompetent to declare whether or not the jest is a good one. He himself must be in a jovial, or at least indifferent, state of mind in order to become the third person of the jest. The same hindrance is present in the case of both harmless and tendency wit; but in the latter the antagonism to the tendency which wishes to serve wit, appears as a new hindrance. The readiness to laugh about an excellent smutty joke cannot manifest itself if the exposure concerns an honored kinsman of the third person. In an assemblage of divines and pastors no one would dare to refer to Heine's comparison of Catholic and Protestant priests as retail dealers and employees of a wholesale business. In the presence of my opponent's friends the wittiest invectives with which I might assail him would not be considered witticisms but invectives, and in the minds of my hearers it would create not pleasure, but indignation. A certain amount of willingness or a certain indifference, the absence of all factors which might evoke strong feelings in opposition to the tendency, are absolute conditions for the participation of the third person in the completion of the wit process.

The Third Person of the Witticism

Wherever such hindrances to the operation of wit fail, we see the phenomenon which we are now investigating, namely, that the pleasure which the wit has provided manifests itself more clearly in the third person than in the

originator of the wit. We must be satisfied to
use the expression " more clearly " where we
should be inclined to ask whether the pleasure
of the hearer is not more intensive than that of
the wit producer, because we are obviously
lacking the means of measuring and comparing
it. We see, however, that the hearer shows his
pleasure by means of explosive laughter after
the first person, in most cases with a serious
expression on his face, has related the joke.
If I repeat a witticism which I have heard, I
am forced, in order not to spoil its effect, to
conduct myself during its recital exactly like
him who made it. We may now put the question whether from this determination of
laughter over wit we can draw conclusions concerning the psychic process of wit-formation.

Now it cannot be our intention to take into
consideration everything that has been asserted
and printed about the nature of laughter. We
are deterred from this undertaking by the
statement which Dugas, one of Ribot's pupils,
put at the beginning of his book *Psychologie
du rire* (1902). " Il n'est pas de fait plus
banal et plus étudié que le rire, il n'en est pas
qui ait eu le don d'exciter davantage la curi-
osité du vulgaire et celle des philosophes, il n'ent
est pas sur lequel on ait recueilli plus d'observations et bâti plus de théories, et avec cela

il n'en est pas qui demeure plus inexpliqué, on serait tenté de dire avec les sceptiques qu'il faut être content de rire et de ne pas chercher à savoir pourquoi on rit, d'autant que peut-être le réflexion tue le rire, et qu'il serait alors contradictoire qu'elle en découvrit les causes" (page 1).

On the other hand, we must make sure to utilize for our purposes a view of the mechanism of laughter which fits our own realm of thought excellently. I refer to the attempted explanation of H. Spencer in his essay entitled *Physiology of Laughter.*[1]

According to Spencer laughter is a phenomenon of discharge of psychic irritation, and an evidence of the fact that the psychic utilization of this irritation has suddenly met with a hindrance. The psychological situation, which discharges itself in laughter, he describes in the following words: "Laughter naturally results only when consciousness is unawares transferred from great things to small—only when there is what we call a descending incongruity."[2]

---

[1] H. Spencer, *The Physiology of Laughter* (first published in *Macmillan's Magazine* for March, 1860), Essays, Vol. 11, 1901.

[2] Different points in this declaration would demand an exhaustive inquiry into an investigation of the pleasure of the comic, a thing that other authors have already done, and which, at all events, does not touch our discussion. It seems to me

In an almost analogous sense the French authors (Dugas) designate laughter as a "détente," a manifestation of release of tension, and A. Bain's theory, "Laughter a relief from restraint," seems to me to approach Spencer's conceptions nearer than many authors would have us believe.

However, we experience the desire to modify Spencer's thought; to give a more definite meaning to some of the ideas and to change others. We would say that laughter arises when the sum total of psychic energy, formerly used for the occupation of certain psychic channels, has become unutilizable so that it can experience absolute discharge. We know what criticism such a declaration invites, but for our

that Spencer was not happy in his explanation of why the discharge happens to find just that path, the excitement of which results in the physical picture of laughter. I should like to add one single contribution to the subject of the physiological explanation of laughter, that is, to the derivation or interpretation of the muscular actions that characterize laughter—a subject that has been often treated before and since Darwin, but which has never been conclusively settled. According to the best of my knowledge the grimaces and contortions of the corners of the mouth that characterize laughter appear first in the satisfied and satiated nursling when he drowsily quits the breasts. There it is a correct motion of expression since it bespeaks the determination to take no more nourishment, an " enough," so to speak, or rather a " more than enough." This primal sense of pleasurable satiation may have furnished the smile, which ever remains the basic phenomenon of laughter, the later connection with the pleasurable processes of discharge.

defense we dare cite a pertinent quotation from Lipps's treatise on *Komik und Humor,* an analysis which throws light on other problems besides the comic and humor. He says: " In the end individual psychological problems always lead us fairly deeply into psychology, so that fundamentally no psychological problem may be considered by itself " (p. 71). The terms " psychic energy," " discharge," and the treatment of psychic energy as a quantity have become habitual modes of thinking since I began to explain to myself the fact of psychopathology philosophically. Being of the same opinion as Lipps I have essayed to represent in my *Interpretation of Dreams* the unconscious psychic processes as real entities, and I have not represented the conscious contents as the " real psychic activity." [1] Only when I speak about the " investing energy (*Besetzung*)

[1] Cf. *The Interpretation of Dreams,* Chap. VII, also *On the Psychic Force,* etc., in the above cited book of Lipps (p. 123), where he says: " This is the general principle: The dominant factors of the psychic life are not represented by the contents of consciousness but by those psychic processes which are unconscious. The task of psychology, provided it does not limit itself to a mere description of the content of consciousness, must also consist of revealing the nature of these unconscious processes from the nature of the contents of consciousness and its temporal relationship. Psychology must itself be a theory of these processes. But such a psychology will soon find that there exist quite a number of characteristics of these processes which are unrepresented in the corresponding contents of consciousness.

of psychic channels," do I seem to deviate from the analogies that Lipps uses. The knowledge that I have gained about the fact that psychic energy can be displaced from one idea to another along certain association channels, and about the almost indestructible conservation of the traces of psychic processes, have actually made it possible for me to attempt such a representation of the unknown. In order to obviate the possibility of a misunderstanding I must add that I am making no attempt to proclaim that cells and fibers, or the neuron system in vogue nowadays, represent these psychic paths, even if such paths would have to be represented by the organic elements of the nervous system in a manner which cannot yet be indicated.

Laughter as a Discharge

Thus, according to our assumption, the conditions for laughter are such that a sum of psychic energy hitherto employed in the occupation of some paths may experience free discharge. And since not all laughter, (but surely the laughter of wit), is a sign of pleasure, we shall be inclined to refer this pleasure to the release of previously existing static energy (*Besetzungsenergie*). When we see

that the hearer of the witticism laughs, while
the creator of the same cannot, then that must
indicate that in the hearer a sum of damming
energy has been released and discharged,
whereas during the wit formation, either in the
release or in the discharge, inhibitions resulted.
One can characterize the psychic process in the
hearer, in the third person of the witticism,
hardly more pointedly than by asserting that
he has bought the pleasure of the witticism
with very little expenditure on his part. One
might say that it is presented to him. The
words of the witticism which he hears necessarily produce in him that idea or thought-connec-
tion whose formation in him was also resisted
by great inner hindrances. He would have
had to make an effort of his own in order to
bring it about spontaneously like the first person, or he would have had to put forth at least
as much psychic expenditure as to equalize the
force of the suppression or repression of the
inhibition. This psychic expenditure he has
saved himself; according to our former discussion (p. 80) we should say that his pleasure
corresponds to this economy. Following our
understanding of the mechanism of laughter
we should be more likely to say that the static
energy utilized in the inhibition has now suddenly become superfluous and neutralized be-

cause a forbidden idea came into existence on the way to auditory perception and is therefore ready to be discharged through laughter. Essentially both statements amount to the same thing, for the economized expenditure corresponds exactly to the now superfluous inhibition. The latter statement is more obvious, for it permits us to say that the hearer of the witticism laughs with the amount of psychic energy which was liberated by the suspension of inhibition energy; that is, he laughs away, as it were, this amount of psychic energy.

Why the First Person Does Not Laugh

If the person in whom the witticism is formed cannot laugh, then it indicates, as we have just remarked, that there is a deviation from the process in the case of the third person which concerns either the suspension of the inhibition energy or the discharge possibility of the same. But the first of the two cases is inconclusive, as we must presently see. The inhibition energy of the first person must have been dissipated, for otherwise there would have been no witticism, the formation of which had to overcome just such a resistance. Otherwise, too, it would have been impossible for the first person to experience the wit-pleasure which the

removal of the inhibition forced us to deduce.
But there remains a second possibility, namely,
that even though he experienced pleasure the
first person cannot laugh, because the possibility of discharge has been disturbed. In the
production of laughter such discharge is essential; an interruption in the possibility of discharge might result from the attachment of
the freed occupation energy to some immediate
endopsychic possibility. It is well that we have
become cognizant of this possibility; we shall
soon pay more attention to it. But with the
wit-maker still another condition leading to the
same result is possible. Perhaps, after all, no
appreciable amount of energy has been liberated, in spite of the successful release of occupation energy. In the first person of the witticism wit-work actually takes place which
must correspond to a certain amount of fresh
psychic expenditure. Thus the first person
contributes the power which removes the inhibitions and which surely results in a gain of
pleasure for himself; in the case of tendency-
wit it is indeed a very big gain, since the fore-
pleasure gained from the wit-work takes upon
itself the further removal of inhibitions. But
the expenditure of the wit-work is, in every
case, derived from the gain which is the result
of the removal of inhibitions; it is the same

expenditure which escapes from the hearer of the witticism. To confirm what was said above it may be added that the witticism loses its laughter effect in the third person as soon as an expenditure of mental work is exacted of him. The allusions of the witticism must be striking, and the omissions easily supplemented; with the awakening of conscious interest in thinking, the effect of the witticism is regularly made impossible. Here lies the real distinction between the witticism and the riddle. It may be that the psychic constellations during wit-work are not at all favorable to the free discharge of the energy gained. We are not here in a position to gain a deeper understanding; our inquiry as to why the third person laughs we have been able to clear up better than the question why the first person does not laugh.

At any rate, if we have well in mind these views about the conditions of laughter and about the psychic process in the third person, we have arrived at a place where we can satisfactorily elucidate an entire series of peculiarities which are familiar in wit, but which have not been understood. Before an amount of interlocked energy, capable of discharge, is to be liberated in the third person, there are several conditions which must be fulfilled or which at least are desirable. 1. It must be definitely established that the third person really produces this expenditure of energy. 2. Care must be taken that when the latter becomes freed that it should find another psychic use instead of offering itself to the motor discharge. 3. It can be of advantage only if the energy to be liberated in the third person is first strengthened and heightened. Certain processes of wit-work which we can gather together under the caption of secondary or auxiliary techniques serve all these purposes.

The first of these conditions determines one of the qualifications of the third person as hearer of the witticism. He must throughout be so completely in psychic harmony with the first person that he makes use of the same inner inhibitions which the wit-work has overcome in the first person. Whoever is focused on smutty jokes will not be able to derive pleasure from clever exhibitionistic wit. Mr. N.'s aggressions will not be understood by uncultured people who are wont to give free rein to their pleasure gained by insulting others. Every witticism thus demands its own public, and to laugh over the same witticisms is a proof of absolute psychic agreement. We have indeed arrived at a point where we are at liberty to examine even more thoroughly the process in the third person's mind. The latter must be able habitually to produce the same inhibition which the joke has surmounted in the first person, so that, as soon as he hears the joke, there awakens within him compulsively and automatically a readiness for this inhibition. This readiness for the inhibition, which I must conceive as a true expenditure analogous to the mobilization.of an army, is simultaneously recognized as superfluous or as belated, and is thus immediately discharged in its nascent state through the channel of laughter.[1]

The second condition for the production of the free discharge, a cutting off of any other outlets for the liberated energy, seems to me of far greater importance. It furnishes the theoretical explanation for the uncertainty of the effect of wit; if the thoughts expressed in the witticism evoke very exciting ideas in the hearer, (depending on the agreement or antagonism between the wit's tendencies and the train of thought dominating the hearer), the witty process either receives or is refused attention. Of still greater theoretical interest, however, are a series of auxiliary wit-techniques which obviously serve the purpose of diverting the attention of the listeners from the

[1] Heymans (*Zeitschrift für Psychol.*, XI) has taken up the viewpoint of the nascent state in a somewhat different connection.

wit-process so as to allow the latter to proceed automatically. I advisedly use the term " automatically " rather than " unconsciously " because the latter designation might prove misleading. It is only a question of keeping the psychic process from getting more than its share of attention during the recital of the witticism, and the usefulness of these auxiliary techniques permits us to assume rightfully that it is just the occupation of attention which has a large share in the control and in the fresh utilization of the freed energv of occupation.

The Automatism of the Wit-process

It seems to be by no means easy to avoid the endopsychic utilization of energy that has become superfluous, for in our mental processes we are constantly in the habit of transferring such emotional outputs from one path to another without losing any of their energy through discharge. Wit prevents this in the following way. In the first place it strives for the shortest possible expression in order te expose less points of attack to the attention. Secondly, it strictly adheres to the condition tnat it be easily understood (v. s.), for as soon as it has recourse to mental effort or demands a choice between different mental paths, it

imperils the effect not only through the un-
avoidable mental expenditure, but also through
the awakening of attention. Besides this, wit
also makes use of the artifice of diverting the
attention by offering to it something in the expression of the witticism which fascinates it so
that meanwhile the liberation of inhibition
energy and its discharge can take place undis-
turbed. The omissions in the wording of wit
already carry out this intention. They impel
us to fill in the gaps and in this way they keep
the wit-process free from attention. The technique of the riddle, as it were, which attracts
attention is here pressed into the service of the
wit-work. The façade formations, which we
have already discovered in many groups of
tendency-wit, are still more effective (see p.
155). The syllogistical façades excellently fulfill the purpose of riveting the attention by an
allotted task. While we begin to ponder
wherein the given answer was lacking already
we are laughing; our attention has been surprised, and the discharge of the liberated emotional inhibition has been effected. The same
is true of witticisms possessing a comic façade
in which the comic serves to assist the wit-
technique. A comic façade promotes the effect of wit in more than one way; it makes
possible not only the automatism of the wit-

process by riveting the attention, but also it facilitates the discharge of wit by sending ahead a discharge from the comic. Here the effect of the comic resembles that of a fascinating fore-pleasure, and we can thus understand that many witticisms are able to dispense entirely the fore-pleasures produced by other means of wit, and make use of only the comic as a fore-pleasure. Among the true techniques of wit it is especially displacement and representation through absurdity which, besides other properties, also develop the deviation of attention so desirable for the automatic discharge of the wit-process.[1]

We already surmise, and later will be able to see more clearly, that in this condition of deviation of attention we have disclosed no un-

---

[1] Through an example of displacement-wit I desire to discuss another interesting character of the technique of wit. The genial actress Gallmeyer when once asked how old she was is said to have answered this unwelcome question with abashed and downcast eyes, by saying, "In Brünn." This is a very good example of displacement. Having been asked her age, she replied by naming the place of her birth, thus anticipating the next query, and in this manner she wishes to imply: "This is a question which I prefer to pass by." And still we feel that the character of the witticism does not here come to expression undimmed. The deviation from the question is too obvious; the displacement is much too conspicuous. Our attention understands immediately that it is a matter of an intentional displacement. In other displacement-witticisms the displacement is disguised and our attention is riveted by the effort to discover it. In one of the displacement-witticisms (p. 69) the reply

essential characteristic of the psychic process in the hearer of wit. In conjunction with this, we can understand something more. First, how it happens that we rarely ever know in a joke why we are laughing, although by analytical investigation we can determine the cause. This laughing is the result of an automatic process which was first made possible by keeping our conscious attention at a distance. Secondly, we arrive at an understanding of that characteristic of wit as a result of which wit can exert its full effect on the hearer only when it is new and when it comes to him as a surprise. This property of wit, which causes wit to be short-lived and forever urges the production of new wit, is evidently due to the fact that it is inherent in the surprising or the unexpected to succeed but once. When we re-

to the recommendation of the horse—" What in the world should I do in Monticello at 6:30 in the morning? "—the displacement is also an obtrusive one, but as a substitute for it it acts upon the attention in a senseless and confusing manner, whereas in the interrogation of the actress we know immediately how to dispose of her displacement answer.

The so-called " facetious questions " which may make use of the best techniques deviate from wit in other ways. An example of the facetious question with displacement is the following: " What is a cannibal who devours his father and mother?—Answer: An orphan.—And when he has devoured all his other relatives?—Sole-heir.—And where can such a monster ever find sympathy?—In the dictionary under S." The facetious questions are not full witticisms because the required witty answers cannot be guessed like the allusions, omissions, etc., of wit.

peat wit the awakened memory leads the attention to the first hearing. This also explains the desire to impart wit to others who have not heard it before, for the impression made by wit on the new hearer replenishes that part of the pleasure which has been lost by the lack of novelty. And an analogous motive probably urges the wit producer to impart his wit to others.

Elements Favoring the Wit-process

As elements favoring the wit-process, even if we can no longer consider them essentials, I present in the third place three technical aids to wit-work which are destined to increase the sums of energy to be discharged and thus enhance the effect of the wit. These technical aids also very often accentuate the attention directed to the wit, but they neutralize its influence by simultaneously fascinating it and impeding its movements. Everything that provokes interest and confusion exerts its influence in these two directions. This is especially true of the nonsense and contrast elements, and above all the "contrast of ideas," which some authors consider the essential character of wit, but in which I see only a means to reinforce the effect of wit. All that is confusing evokes in the hearer that condition of distribution of energy which Lipps has designated as " psychic damming "; and, doubtless, he has a right to assume that the force of the " discharge " varies with the success of the damming process which precedes it. Lipps's exposition does not explicitly refer to wit, but to the comic in general, yet it seems quite probable that the discharge in wit, releasing a gush of inhibition energy, is brought to its height in a similar manner by means of the damming.

At length we are aware that the technique of wit is really determined by two kinds of tendencies, those which make possible the formation of wit in the first person, and those guaranteeing that the witticism produces in the third person as much pleasurable effect as possible. The Janus-like double-facedness of wit, which safeguards its original resultant pleasure against the impugnment of critical reason, belongs to the first tendency together with the mechanism of fore-pleasure; the other complications of technique produced by the conditions discussed in this chapter concern the third person of the witticism. Thus wit in itself is a double-tongued villain which serves two masters at the same time. Everything that aims toward gaining pleasure is calculated by the witticism to arouse the third person, as if inner, unsurmountable inhibitions in the first person were in the way of the same. Thus one gets the full impression of the absolute necessity of this third person for the completion of the wit-process. But while we have succeeded in obtaining a good insight concerning the nature of this process in the third person, we feel that the corresponding process in the first person is still shrouded in darkness. So far we have not succeeded in answering the first of our two questions: Why can we not laugh over wit made by ourselves? and: Why are we urged to impart our own witticisms to others? We can only suspect that there is an intimate connection between the two facts yet to be explained, and that we must impart our witticisms to others for the reason that we ourselves are unable to laugh over them. From our examinations of the conditions in the third person for pleasure gaining and pleasure discharging we can draw the conclusion that in the first person the conditions for discharge are lacking and that those for gaining pleasure are only incompletely fulfilled. Thus it is not to be disputed that we enhance our pleasure in that we attain the—to us impossible— laughter in this roundabout way from the impression of the person who was stimulated to laughter. Thus we laugh, so to speak, *par ricochet,* as Dugas expresses it. Laughter belongs to those manifestations of psychic states which are highly infectious; if I make some one else laugh by imparting my wit to him, I am really using him as a tool in order to arouse my own laughter. One can really notice that the person who at first recites the witticism with a serious mien later joins the hearer with a moderate amount of laughter. Imparting my witticisms to others may thus serve several purposes. First, it serves to give me the objective certainty of the success of the wit-work; secondly, it serves to enhance my own pleasure through the reaction of the hearer upon myself; thirdly, in the case of repeating a not original joke, it serves to remedy the loss of pleasure due to the lack of novelty.

Economy and Full Expenditure

At the end of these discussions about the psychic processes of wit, in so far as they are enacted between two persons, we can glance back to the factor of economy which impressed us as an important item in the psychological conception of wit since we offered the first explanation of wit-technique. Long ago we dismissed the nearest but also the simplest conception of this economy, where it was a matter

of avoiding psychic expenditure in general by
a maximum restriction in the use of words and
by the production of associations of ideas. We
had then already asserted that brevity and
laconisms are not witty in themselves. The
brevity of wit is a peculiar one; it has to be
a "witty" brevity. The original pleasure
gain produced by playing with words and
thoughts resulted, to be sure, from simple
economy in expenditure, but with the development of play into wit the tendency to economize also had to shift its goals, for whatever
might be saved by the use of the same words
or by avoiding new thought connections would
surely be of no account when compared to the
colossal expenditure of our mental activity.
We may be permitted to make a comparison
between the psychic economy and a business
enterprise. So long as the latter's transactions
are very small, good policy demands that expenses be kept low and that the costs of operation be minimized as much as possible.
The economy still follows the absolute height
of the expenditure. Later on when the volume of business has increased, the importance
of the business expenses dwindles; increases in
the expenditure totals matter little so long as
the transactions and returns can be sufficiently
increased. Keeping down running expenses

would be parsimonious; in fact, it would mean a direct loss. Nevertheless it would be equally false to assume that with a very great expenditure there would be no more room for saving. The manager inclined to economize would now make an effort to save on particular things and would feel satisfied if the same establishment, with its costly upkeep, could reduce its expenses at all, no matter how small the saving would seem in comparison to the entire expenditure. In quite an analogous manner the detailed economy in our complicated psychic affairs remains a source of pleasure, as may be shown by everyday occurrences. Whoever used to have a gas lamp in his room, but now uses electric light, will experience for a long time a definite feeling of pleasure when he presses the electric light button; this pleasure continues as long as at that moment he remembers the complicated arrangements necessary to light the gas lamp. Similarly the economy of expenditure in psychic inhibition brought about by wit—small though it may be in comparison to the sum total of psychic expenditure—will remain a source of pleasure for us, because we thereby save a particular expenditure which we were wont to make and which as before we were ready to make. That the expenditure is expected and prepared for is a factor which stands unmistakably in the foreground.

A localized economy, as the one just considered, will not fail to give us momentary pleasure, but it will not bring about a lasting alleviation so long as what has been saved here can be utilized in another place. Only when this disposal into a different path can be avoided, will the special economy be transformed into a general alleviation of the psychic expenditures. Thus, with clearer insight into the psychic processes of wit, we see that the factor of alleviation takes the place of economy. Obviously the former gives us the greater feeling of pleasure. The process in the first person of the witticism produces pleasure by removing inhibitions and by diminishing local expenditure; it does not, however, seem to come to rest until it succeeds through the intervention of the third person in attaining general relief through discharge.

C. THEORETICAL PART

VI.

AT the end of the chapter which dealt with
the elucidation of the technique of wit (p. 125)
we asserted that the processes of condensation
with and without substitutive formation, displacement, representation through absurdity,
representation through the opposite, indirect
representation, etc., all of which we found participated in the formation of wit, evinced a
far-reaching agreement with the processes of
" dream-work." We promised, at that time,
first to examine more carefully these similarities, and secondly, so far as such indications
point to search for what is common to both wit
and dreams. The discussion of this comparison would be much easier for us if we could
assume that one of the subjects to be compared—the " dream-work "—were well known.
But we shall probably do better not to take
this assumption for granted. I received the
impression that my book *The Interpretation
of Dreams* created more " confusion " than
" enlightenment " among my colleagues, and I

know that the wider reading circles have contented themselves to reduce the contents of the book to a catchword, " Wish fulfillment " —a term easily remembered and easily abused.

However, in my continued occupation with the problems considered therein, for the study of which my practice as a psychotherapeutist affords me much opportunity, I found nothing that would impel me to change or improve on my ideas; I can therefore peacefully wait until the reader's comprehension has risen to my level, or until an intelligent critic has pointed out to me the basic faults in my conception. For the purposes of comparison with wit, I shall briefly review the most important features of dreams and dream-work.

We know dreams by the recollection which usually seems fragmentary and which occurs upon awakening. It is then a structure made up mostly of visual or other sensory impressions, which represents to us a deceptive picture of an experience, and may be mingled with mental processes (the " knowledge " in the dream) and emotional manifestations. What we thus remember as a dream I call " the manifest dream-content." The latter is often altogether absurd and confused, at other times it is merely one part or another that is so affected. But even if it be entirely coherent,

as in the case of some anxiety dreams, it stands
out in our psychic life as something strange,
for the origin of which one cannot account.
Until recently the explanation for these peculiarities of the dream has been sought in the
dream itself in that it was considered roughly
speaking an indication of a muddled, dissociated, and " sleepy " activity of the nervous elements.

As opposed to this view I have shown that
the excessively peculiar " manifest " dream-
content can regularly be made comprehensible,
and that it is a disfigured and changed
transcription of certain correct psychic formations which deserve the name of " latent dream-
thoughts." One gains an understanding of
the latter by resolving the manifest dream-content into its component parts without regard
for its apparent meaning, and then by following up the threads of associations which emanate from each one of the now isolated elements. These become interwoven and in the
end lead to a structure of thoughts, which is
not only entirely accurate, but also fits easily
into the familiar associations of our psychic
processes. During this " analysis " the dream-
content loses all of the peculiarities so strange
to us; but if the analysis is to be successful,
we must firmly cast aside the critical objections

which incessantly arise against the reproduction of the individual associations.

The Dream-work

From the comparison of the remembered manifest dream-content with the latent dream-thoughts thus discovered there arises the conception of " dream-work." The entire sum of the transforming processes which have changed the latent dream-thought into the manifest dream is called the dream-work. The astonishment which formerly the dream evoked in us is now perceived to be due to the dream-work.

The function of the dream-work may be described in the following manner. A structure of thoughts, mostly very complicated, which has been built up during the day and not brought to settlement—a day remnant—clings firmly even during night to the energy which it had assumed—the underlying center of interest—and thus threatens to disturb sleep. This day remnant is transformed into a dream by the dream-work and in this way rendered harmless to sleep. But in order to make possible its employment by the dream-work, this day remnant must be capable of being cast into the form of a wish, a condition that is not

difficult to fulfill. The wish emanating from
the dream-thoughts forms the first step and
later on the nucleus of the dream. Experience
gained from analyses—not the theory of the
dream—teaches us that with children a fond
wish left from the waking state suffices to
evoke a dream, which is coherent and senseful,
but almost always short, and easny recognizable as a "wish fulfillment." In the case of
adults the universally valid condition for the
dream-creating wish seems to be that the latter
should appear foreign to conscious thinking,
that is, it should be a repressed wish, or that
it should supply consciousness with reinforcement from unknown sources. Without the assumption of the unconscious activity in the
sense used above, I should be at a loss to develop further the theory of dreams and to explain the material gleaned from experience in
dream-analyses. The action of this unconscious
wish upon the logical conscious material of
dream-thoughts now results in the dream. The
latter is thereby drawn down into the unconscious, as it were, or to speak more precisely,
it is exposed to a treatment which usually
takes place at the level of unconscious mental
activity, and which is characteristic of this
mental level. Only from the results of the
"dream-work" have we thus far learned to

know the qualities of this unconscious mental activity and its differentiation from the "fore-conscious" which is capable of consciousness.

The Unconscious

A novel and difficult theory that runs counter to our habitual modes of thinking can hardly gain in lucidity by a condensed exposition. I can therefore accomplish little more in this discussion than refer the reader to the detailed treatment of the unconscious in my *Interpretation of Dreams,* and also to Lipps's work, which I consider most important. I am aware that he who is under the spell of a good old philosophical training, or stands aloof from a so-called philosophical system, will oppose the assumption of the "unconscious psychic processes" in Lipps's sense and in mine and will desire to prove the impossibility of it preferably by means of definitions of the term psychic. But definitions are conventional and changeable. I have often found that persons who dispute the unconscious on the grounds of its absurdity or impossibility have not received their impressions from those sources from which I, at least, have found it necessary to draw, in order to become aware of its existence. These opponents had never witnessed the effect of a posthypnotic suggestion, and they were immensely surprised at the evidence I imparted to them gleaned from my analysis of unhypnotized neurotics. They had never gained the conception of the unconscious as something which one does not really know, while cogent proofs force one to supplement this idea by saying that one understands by the unconscious something capable of consciousness, something concerning which one has not thought and which is not in the field of vision of consciousness. Nor had they attempted to convince themselves of the existence of such unconscious thoughts in their own psychic life by means of an analysis of one of their own dreams, and when I attempted this with them, they could perceive their own mental occurrences only with astonishment and confusion. I have also gotten the impression that these are essentially affective resistances which stand in the way of the acceptation of the " unconscious," and that they are based on the fact that no one is desirous of becoming acquainted with his unconscious, and it is most convenient to deny altogether its possibility.

Condensation and Displacement in the Dream-work

The dream-work, to which I return after this digression, subjects the thought material uttered in the optative mood to a very peculiar elaboration. First of all it proceeds from the optative to the indicative mood; it substitutes " it is " for " would it were! " This " it is " is destined to become part of an hallucinatory representation which I have called the " regression " of the dream-work. This regression represents the path from the mental images to the sensory perceptions of the same, or if one chooses to speak with reference to the still unfamiliar—not to be understood anatomically—topic of the psychic apparatus, it is the region of the thought-formation to the region of the sensory perception. Along this road which runs in an opposite direction to the course of development of psychic complications the dream-thoughts gain in clearness; a plastic situation finally results as a nucleus of the manifest " dream picture." In order to arrive at such a sensory representation the dream-thoughts have had to experience tangible changes in their expression. But while the thoughts are changed back into mental images they are subjected to still greater changes,

some of which are easily conceivable as necessary, while others are surprising. As a necessary secondary result of the regression one
understands that nearly all relationships within
the thoughts which have organized the same
are lost to the manifest dream. The dream-
work takes over, as it were, only the raw material of the ideas for representation, and not
the thought-relations which held each other in
check; or at least it reserves the freedom of
leaving the latter out of the question. On the
other hand, there is a certain part of the dream-
work which cannot be traced to the regression
or to the recasting into mental images; it is
just that part which is significant to us for the
analogy to wit-formation. The material of the
dream-thoughts experiences an extraordinary
compression or *condensation* during the dream-
work. The starting-points of this condensation are those points which are common to two
or more dream-thoughts because they naturally
pertain to both or because they are inevitable
consequences of the contents of two or more
dream-thoughts, and since these points do not
regularly suffice for a prolific condensation
new artificial and fleeting common points come
into existence, and for this purpose preferably
words are used which combine different meanings in their sounds. The newly framed com-

mon points of condensation enter as represent-
atives of the dream-thoughts into the manifest
dream-content, so that an element of the dream
corresponds to a point of junction or intersec-
tion of the dream-thoughts, and with regard
to the latter it must in general be called " over-
determined." The process of condensation is
that part of the dream-work which is most
easily recognizable; it suffices to compare the
recorded wording of a dream with the written
dream-thoughts gained by means of analysis,
in order to get a good impression of the pro-
ductiveness of dream condensation.

It is not easy to convince one's self of the
second great change that takes place in the
dream-thoughts through the agency of the
dream-work. I refer to that process which I
have called the dream *displacement*. It manifests itself by the fact that what occupies the
center of the manifest dream and is endowed
with vivid sensory intensity has occupied a
peripheral and secondary position in the dream-
thoughts, and *vice versa*. This process causes
the dream to appear out of proportion when
compared with the dream-thoughts, and it is
because of this displacement that it seems
strange and incomprehensible to the waking
state. In order that such a displacement
should occur it must be possible for the occu-

pation energy to pass uninhibited from important to insignificant ideas,—a process which in normal conscious thinking can only give the impression of "faulty thinking."

Transformation into expressive activity, condensation, and displacement are the three great functions which we can ascribe to the dream-work. A fourth, to which too little attention was given in *The Interpretation of Dreams,* does not come into consideration here for our purpose. In a consistent elucidation of the ideas dealing with the "topic of the psychic apparatus" and "regression," which alone can lend value to these working hypotheses, an effort would have to be made to determine at what stages of regression the various transformations of the dream-thoughts occur. As yet no serious effort has been made in this direction, but at least we can speak definitely about displacement when we say that it must arise in the thought material while the latter is in the level of the unconscious processes. One will probably have to think of condensation as a process that extends over the entire course up to the outposts of the perceptive region; but in general it suffices to assume that there is a simultaneous activity of all the forces which participate in the formation of dreams. In view of the reserve which one must

naturally exercise in the treatment of such
problems, and in consideration of the inability
to discuss here the main objections to these
problems, I should like to trust somewhat to
the assertion that the process of the dream-
work which prepares the dream is situated in
the region of the unconscious. Roughly speaking, one can distinguish three general stages
in the formation of the dream: first, the transference of the conscious day remnants into the
unconscious, a transference in which the conditions of the sleeping state must co-operate;
secondly, the actual dream-work in the
unconscious; and thirdly, the regression of
the elaborated dream material to the region
of perception, whereby the dream becomes
conscious.

The forces participating in the dream-formation may be recognized as the following: the
wish to sleep; the sum of occupation energy
which still clings to the day remnants after the
depression brought about by the state of sleep;
the psychic energy of the unconscious wish
forming the dream; and the opposing force of
the " censor," which exercises its authority in
our waking state, and is not entirely abolished
during sleep. The task of dream-formation is,
above all, to overcome the inhibition of the
censor, and it is just this task that is fulfilled

by the displacement of the psychic energy within the material of the dream-thoughts.

The Formula for Wit-work

Now we recall what caused us to think of the dream while investigating wit. We found that the character and activity of wit were bound up in cèrtain forms of expression and technical means, among which the various forms of condensation, displacement, and indirect representation were the most conspicuous. But the processes which led to the same results —condensation, displacement, and indirect expression—we learned to know as peculiarities of dream-work. Does not this analogy almost force us to the conclusion that wit-work and dream-work must be identical at least in one essential point? I believe that the dream-work lies revealed before us in its most important characters, but in wit we find obscured just that portion of the psychic processes which we may compare with the dream-work, namely, the process of wit-formation in the first person. Shall we not yield to the temptation to construct this process according to the analogy of dream-formation? Some of the characteristics of dreams are so foreign to wit that that part of the dream-work corresponding to them cannot be carried over to the wit-formation. The regression of the stream of thought to perception certainly falls away as far as wit is concerned. However, the other two stages of dream-formation, the sinking of a foreconscious [1] thought into the unconscious, and the unconscious elaboration, would give us exactly the result which we might observe in wit if we assumed this process in wit-formation. Let us decide to assume that this is the proceeding of wit-formation in the case of the first person. *A foreconscious thought is left for a moment to unconscious elaboration and the results are forthwith grasped by the conscious perception.*

Before, however, we attempt to prove the details of this assertion we wish to consider an objection which may jeopardize our assumption. We start with the fact that the techniques of wit point to the same processes which become known to us as peculiarities of dream-work. Now it is an easy matter to say in opposition that we would not have described the techniques of wit as condensation, displacement, etc., nor would we have arrived at such a comprehensive agreement in the means of representation of wit and dreams, if our previous knowledge of dream-work had not influenced our conception of the technique of wit; so that

[1] Cf. *The Interpretation of Dreams*, Chapter VII.

at the bottom we find that wit confirms only those tentative theories which we brought to it from our study of dreams. Such a genesis of ł greement would be no certain guarantee of its tability beyond our preconceived judgment. No other author has thought of considering condensation, displacement, and indirect expression as active factors of wit. This might be a possible objection, but nevertheless it would not be justified. It might just as well be said that in order to recognize the real agreement between dreams and wit our ordinary knowledge must be augmented by a specialized knowledge of dream-work. However, the decision will really depend only upon the question whether the examining critic can prove that such a conception of the technique of wit in the individual examples is forced, and that other nearer and farther-reaching interpretations have been suppressed in favor of mine; or whether the critic will have to admit that the tentative theories derived from the study of dreams can be really confirmed through wit. My opinion is that we have nothing to fear from such a critic and that our processes of reduction have confidently pointed out in which forms of expression we must search for the techniques of wit. That we designated these techniques by names which previously anticipated the result of the agreement between the technique of wit and the dream-work was our just prerogative, and really nothing more than an easily justified simplification.

There is still another objection which would not be vital, but which could not be so completely refuted. One might think that the techniques of wit that fit in so well considering the ends we have in view deserve recognition, but that they do not represent all possible techniques of wit or even all those in use. Also that we have selected only the techniques of wit which were influenced by and would suit the pattern of the dream-work, whereas others ignored by us would have demonstrated that such an agreement was not common to all cases. I really do not trust myself to make the assertion that I have succeeded in explaining all the current witticisms with reference to their techniques, and I therefore admit the possibility that my enumeration of wit-techniques may show many gaps. But I have not purposely excluded from my discussion any form of technique that was clear to me, and I can affirm that the most frequent, the most essential, and the most characteristic technical means of wit have not eluded my attention.

Wit as an Inspiration

Wit possesses still another character which entirely corresponds to our conception of the wit-work as originally discovered in our study of dreams. It is true that it is common to hear one say " I *made* a joke," but one feels that one behaves differently during this process than when one pronounces a judgment or offers an objection. Wit shows in a most pronounced manner the character of an involuntary " inspiration " or a sudden flash of thought. A moment before one cannot tell what kind of joke one is going to make, though it lacks only the words to clothe it. One usually experiences something indefinable which I should like most to compare to an absence, or sudden drop of intellectual tension; then all of a sudden the witticism appears, usually simultaneously with its verbal investment. Some of the means of wit are also utilized in the expression of thought along other lines, as in the cases of comparison and allusion. I can purposely will to make an allusion. In doing this I have first in mind (in the inner hearing) the direct expression of my thought, but as I am inhibited from expressing the same through some objection from the situation in question, I almost resolve to substitute the direct expression by a form of indirect expression, and then I utter it in the form of an allusion. But the allusion that comes into existence in this manner having been formed under my continuous control is never witty, no matter how useful it may be. On the other hand, the witty allusion appears without my having been able to follow up these preparatory stages in my mind. I do not wish to attribute too much value to this procedure, it is scarcely decisive, but it does agree well with our assumption that in wit-formation a stream of thought is dropped for a moment and suddenly emerges from the unconscious as a witticism.

Witticisms also evince a peculiar behavior along the lines of association of ideas. Frequently they are not at the disposal of our memory when we look for them; on the other hand, they often appear unsolicited and at places in our train of thought where we cannot understand their presence. Again, these are only minor qualities, but none the less they point to their unconscious origin.

Let us now collect the properties of wit whose formation can be referred to the unconscious. Above all there is the peculiar brevity of wit which, though not an indispensable, is a marked and distinctive characteristic feature.

When we first encountered it we were inclined to see in it an expression of a tendency to economize, but owing to very evident objections we ourselves depreciated the value of this conception. At present we look upon it more as a sign of the unconscious elaboration which the thought of wit has undergone. The process of condensation which corresponds to it in dreams we can correlate with no other factor than with the localization in the unconscious, and we must assume that the conditions for such condensations which are lacking in the foreconscious are present in the unconscious mental process.[1] It is to be expected that in the process of condensation some of the elements subjected to it become lost, while others which take over their occupation energy are strengthened by the condensation or are built up too energetically. The brevity of wit, like the brevity of dreams, would thus be a necessary concomitant manifestation of the con densation which occurs in both cases; both times it is a result of the condensation process.

[1] Besides the dream-work and the technique of wit I have been able to demonstrate condensation as a regular and significant process in another psychic occurrence, in the mechanism of normal (not purposive) forgetting. Singular impressions put difficulties in the way of forgetting; impressions in any way analogous are forgotten by becoming fused at their points of contact. The confusion of analogous impressions is one of the first steps in forgetting.

The brevity of wit is indebted also to this origin for its peculiar character which though not further assignable produces a striking impression.

The Unconscious and the Infantile.

We have defined above the one result of condensation—the manifold application of the same material, play upon words, and similarity of sound—as a localized economy, and have also referred the pleasure produced by harmless wit to that economy. At a later place we have found that the original purpose of wit consisted in producing this kind of pleasure from words, a process which was permitted to the individual during the stage of playing, but which became banked in during the course of intellectual development or by rational criticism. Now we have decided upon the assumption that such condensations as serve the technique of wit originate automatically and without any particular purpose during the process of thinking in the unconscious. Have we not here two different conceptions of the same fact which seem to be incompatible with each other? I do not think so. To be sure, there are two different conceptions, and they demand to be brought in unison, but they do not contradict

each other. They are merely somewhat
strange to each other, and as soon as we have
established a relationship between them we
shall probably gain in knowledge. That such
condensations are sources of pleasure is in perfect accord with the supposition that they
easily find in the unconscious the conditions
necessary for their origin; on the other hand,
we see the motivation for the sinking into the
unconscious in the circumstance that the pleasure-bringing condensation necessary to wit
easily results there. Two other factors also,
which upon first examination seem entirely
foreign to each other and which are brought
together quite accidentally, will be recognized on deeper investigation as intimately
connected, and perhaps may be found to
be substantially the same. I am referring
to the two assertions that on the one hand
wit could form such pleasure-bringing condensations during its development in the stage
of playing, that is, during the infancy of reason; and, on the other hand, that it accomplishes the same function on higher levels by
submerging the thought into the unconscious.
For the infantile is the source of the unconscious. The unconscious mental processes are
no others than those which are solely produced
during infancy. The thought which sinks into

the unconscious for the purpose of wit-formation only revisits there the old homestead of the former playing with words. The thought is put back for a moment into the infantile state in order to regain in this way childish pleasure-sources. If, indeed, one were not already acquainted with it from the investigation of the psychology of the neuroses, wit would surely impress one with the idea that the peculiar unconscious elaboration is nothing else but the infantile type of the mental process. Only it is by no means an easy matter to grasp, in the unconscious of the adult, this peculiar infantile manner of thinking, because it is usually corrected, so to say, *statu nascendi*. However, it is successfully grasped in a series of cases, and then we always laugh about the " childish stupidity." In fact every exposure of such an unconscious fact affects us in a " comical " manner.[1]

It is easier to comprehend the character of these unconscious mental processes in the utterances of patients suffering from various psy-

[1] Many of my patients while under psychoanalytic treatment are wont to prove regularly by their laughter that I have succeeded in demonstrating faithfully to their conscious perception the veiled unconscious; they laugh also when the content of what is disclosed does not at all justify this laughter. To be sure, it is conditional that they have approached this unconscious closely enough to grasp it when the physician has conjectured it and presented it to them.

chic disturbances. It is very probable that, following the assumption of old Griesinger, we would be in a position to understand the deliria of the insane and to turn them to good account as valuable information, if we would not make the demands of conscious thinking upon them, but instead treat them as we do dreams by means of our art of interpretation.[1] In the dream, too, we were able to show the " return of psychic life to the embryonal state." [2]

In discussing the processes of condensation we have entered so deeply into the signification of the analogy between wit and dreams that we can here be brief. As we know that displacements in dream-work point to the influence of the censor of conscious thought, we will consequently be inclined to assume that an inhibiting force also plays a part in the formation of wit when we find the process of displacement among the techniques of wit. We also know that this is commonly the case; the endeavor of wit to revive the old pleasure in nonsense or the old pleasure in word-play meets with resistance in every normal state, a resistance which is exerted by the protest of critical reason, and which must be overcome in each in-

---

[1] In doing this we must not forget to reckon with the distortion brought about by the censor which is still active in the psychoses.

[2] *The Interpretation of Dreams.*

dividual case. But a radical distinction between wit and dreams is shown in the manner in which the wit-work solves this difficulty. In the dream-work the solution of this task is brought about regularly through displacements and through the choice of ideas which are remote enough from the objectionable ones to secure passage through the censor; the latter themselves are but offsprings of those whose psychic energy they have taken upon themselves through full transference. The displacements are therefore not lacking in any dream and are far more comprehensive; they not only comprise the deviations from the trend of thought but also all forms of indirect expression, the substitution for an important but offensive element of one seemingly indifferent and harmless to the censor which form very remote allusions to the first, they include substitution also occurring through symbols, comparisons, or trifles. It is not to be denied that parts of this indirect representation really originate in the foreconscious thoughts of the dream,—as, for example, symbolical representation and representation through comparisons—because otherwise the thought would not have reached the state of the foreconscious expression. Such indirect expressions and allusions, whose reference to the original thought is easily findable, are really permissible and customary means of expression even in our conscious thought. The dream-work, however, exaggerates the application of these means of indirect expression to an unlimited degree. Under the pressure of the censor any kind of association becomes good enough for substitution by allusion; the displacement from one element to any other is permitted. The substitution of the inner associations (similarity, causal connection, etc.) by the so-called outer associations (simultaneity, contiguity in space, assonance) is particularly conspicuous and characteristic of the dream-work.

The Difference between Dream-technique and Wit-technique

All these means of displacement also occur as techniques of wit, but when they do occur they usually restrict themselves to those limits prescribed for their use in conscious thought; in fact they may be lacking, even though wit must regularly solve a task of inhibition. One can comprehend this retirement of the process of displacement in wit-work when one remembers that wit usually has another technique at its disposal through which it defends itself against inhibitions. Indeed, we have discovered nothing more characteristic of it than just this technique. For wit does not have recourse to compromises as does the dream, nor does it evade the inhibition; it insists upon retaining the play with words or nonsense unaltered, but thanks to the ambiguity of words and multiplicity of thought-relations, it restricts itself to the choice of cases in which this play or nonsense may appear at the same time admissible (jest) or senseful (wit). Nothing distinguishes wit from all other psychic formations better than this double-sidedness and this double-dealing; by emphasizing the " sense in nonsense," the authors have approached nearest the understanding of wit, at least from this angle.

Considering the unexceptional predominance of this peculiar technique in overcoming inhibitions in wit, one might find it superfluous that wit should make use of the displacement-technique even in a single case. But on the one hand certain kinds of this technique remain useful for wit as objects and sources of pleasure—as, for example, the real displacement (deviation of the trend of thought) which in fact shares in the nature of nonsense,—and on the other hand one must not forget that the highest stage of wit, tendency-wit, must frequently overcome two kinds of inhibitions which oppose both itself and its tendency (p. 147), and that allusion and displacements are qualified to facilitate this latter task.

The numerous and unrestricted application of indirect representation, of displacements, and especially of allusions in the dream-work, has a result which I mention not because of its own significance but because it became for me the subjective inducement to occupy myself with the problem of wit. If a dream analysis is imparted to one unfamiliar with the subject and unaccustomed to it, and the peculiar ways of allusions and displacements (objectionable to the waking thoughts but utilized by the dream-work) are explained, the hearer experiences an uncomfortable impression; he declares these interpretations to be "witty," but it seems obvious to him that these are not successful jokes but forced ones which run contrary to the rules of wit. This impression can be easily explained; it is due to the fact that the dream-work operates with the same means as wit, but in the application of the same the dream exceeds the bounds which wit restricts. We shall soon learn that in consequence of the rôle of the third person wit is bound by a certain condition which does not affect the dream.

Irony—Negativism.

Among those techniques which are common to both wit and dreams representation through the opposite and the application of absurdity are especially interesting. The first belongs to the strongly effective means of wit as shown in the examples of " out-doing wit " (p. 98). The representation through the opposite, unlike most of the wit-techniques, is unable to withdraw itself from conscious attention. He who intentionally tries to make use of wit-work, as in the case of the " habitual wit," soon discovers that the easiest way to answer an assertion with a witticism is to concentrate one's mind on the opposite of this assertion and trust to the chance flash of thought to brush aside the feared objection to this opposite by means of a different interpretation. Maybe the representation through its opposite is indebted for such a preference to the fact that it forms the nucleus of another pleasurable mode of mental expression, for an understanding of which we do not have to consult the unconscious. I refer to *irony,* which is very similar to wit and is considered a sub-species of the comic. The essence of irony consists in imparting the very opposite of what one intended to express, but it precludes the anticipated contradiction by indicating through the inflections, concomitant gestures, and through slight changes in style—if it is done in writing—that the speaker himself means to convey the opposite of what he says. Irony is applicable only in cases where the other person is prepared to hear the reverse of the statement actually made, so that he cannot fail to be inclined to contradict. As a consequence of this condition ironic expressions are particularly subject to the danger of being misunderstood. To the person who uses it, it gives the advantage of readily avoiding the difficulties to which direct expressions, as, for example, invectives, are subject. In the hearer it produces comic pleasure, probably by causing him to make preparations for contradiction, which are immediately found to be unnecessary. Such a comparison of wit with a form of the comical that is closely allied to it might strengthen us in the assumption that the relation of wit to the unconscious is the peculiarity that also distinguishes it from the comical.[1]

In dream-work, representation through the opposite has a far more important part to play than in wit. The dream not only delights in

[1] The character of the comical which is referred to as its "dryness" also depends in the broadest sense upon the differentiation of the things spoken from the antics accompanying it.

representing a pair of opposites by means of
one and the same composite image, but in addition it often changes an element from the
dream-thoughts into its opposite, thus causing
considerable difficulty in the work of interpretation. In the case of any element capable of
having an opposite it is impossible to tell
whether it is to be taken negatively or positively in the dream-thoughts.[1]

I must emphasize that as yet this fact has
by no means been understood. Nevertheless,
it seems to give indications of an important
characteristic of unconscious thinking which in
all probability results in a process comparable
to " judging." Instead of setting aside judgments the unconscious forms " repressions."
The repression may correctly be described as
a stage intermediate between the defense reflex and condemnation.[2]

---

[1] *The Interpretation of Dreams*, p. 296.

[2] This very remarkable and still inadequately understood behavior of antagonistic relationships is probably not without value
for the understanding of the symptom of negativism in neurotics
and in the insane. Cf. the two latest works on the subject: Bleu-
ler, " Über die negative Suggestibilität," *Psych.-Neurol. Wochen-
schrift*, 1904, and Otto Groos's *Zur Differential diagnostik nega-
tivistischer Phänomene*, also my review of the *Gegensinn der
Urworte*, in *Jahrb. f. Psychonalyse* II, 1910.

The Unconscious as the Psychic Stage of the Wit-work

Nonsense, or absurdity, which occurs so often in dreams and which has made them the object of so much contempt, has never really come into being as the result of an accidental shuffling of conceptual elements, but may in every case be proven to have been purposely admitted by the dream-work. Nonsense and absurdity are intended to express embittered criticism and scornful contradiction within the dream-thoughts. Absurdity in the dream-content thus stands for the judgment: " It's pure nonsense," expressed in dream-thoughts. In my work on the Interpretation of Dreams, I have placed great emphasis on the demonstration of this fact because I thought that I could in this manner most strikingly controvert the error expressed by many that the dream is no psychic phenomenon at all—an error which bars the way to an understanding of the unconscious. Now we have learnt (in the analysis of certain tendency-witticisms on p. 73). that nonsense in wit is made to serve the same purposes of expression. We also know that a nonsensical façade of a witticism is peculiarly adapted to enhance the psychic expenditure in the hearer and hence also to increase the amount to be discharged through laughter. Moreover, we must not forget that nonsense in wit is an end in itself, since the purpose of reviving the old pleasure in nonsense is one of the motives of the wit-work. There are other ways to regain the feeling of nonsense in order to derive pleasure from it; caricature, exaggeration, parody, and travesty utilize the same and thus produce "comical nonsense." If we subject these modes of expression to an analysis similar to the one used in studying wit, we shall find that there is no occasion in any of them for resorting to unconscious processes in our sense for the purpose of getting explanations. We are now also in a position to understand why the "witty" character may be added as an embellishment to caricature, exaggeration, and parody; it is the manifold character of the performance upon the "psychic stage"[1] that makes this possible.

I am of the opinion that by transferring the wit-work into the system of the unconscious we have made a distinct gain, since it makes it possible for us to understand the fact that the various techniques to which wit admittedly adheres are on the other hand not its exclusive

[1] An expression of G. T. Fechner's which has acquired significance from the point of view of my conception.

property. Many doubts, which have arisen in the beginning of our investigation of these techniques and which we were forced temporarily to leave, can now be conveniently cleared up. Hence we shall give due consideration to the doubt which expresses itself by asserting that the undeniable relation of wit to the unconscious is correct only for certain categories of tendency-wit, while we are ready to claim this relation for all forms and all the stages of development of wit. We may not shirk the duty of testing this objection.

We may assume that we deal with a sure case of wit-formation in the unconscious when it concerns witticisms that serve unconscious tendencies, or those strengthened by unconscious tendencies, as, for example, most "cynical" witticisms. For in such cases the unconscious tendency draws the foreconscious thought down into the unconscious in order to remodel it there; a process to which the study of the psychology of the neuroses has added many analogies with which we are acquainted. But in the case of tendency-wit of other varieties, namely, harmless wit and the jest, this power seems to fall away, and the relation of the wit to the unconscious is an open question.

But now let us consider the case of the witty expression of a thought that is not without value in itself and that comes to the surface in the course of the association of mental processes. In order that this thought may become a witticism, it is of course necessary that it make a choice among the possible forms of expression in order to find the exact form that will bring along the gain in word-pleasure. We know from self-observation that this choice is not made by conscious attention; but the selection will certainly be better if the occupation energy of the foreconscious thought is lowered to the unconscious. For in the unconscious, as we have learnt from the dream-work, the paths of association emanating from a word are treated on a par with associations from objects. The occupation energy from the unconscious presents by far the more favorable conditions for the selection of the expression. Moreover, we may assume without going farther that the possible expression which contains the gain in word-pleasure exerts a lowering effect on the still fluctuating self-command of the foreconscious, similar to that exerted in the first case by the unconscious tendency. As an explanation for the simpler case of the jest we may imagine that an ever-watchful intention of attaining the gain in word-pleasure seizes the opportunity offered in the foreconscious of again drawing the in vesting energy down into the unconscious, according to the familiar scheme.

I earnestly wish that it were possible for me on the one hand to present one decisive point in my conception of wit more clearly, and on the other hand to fortify it with compelling arguments. But as a matter of fact it is not a question here of two failures, but of one and the same failure. I can give no clearer exposition because I have no further testimony on behalf of my conception. The latter has developed as the result of my study of the technique and of comparison with dream-work, and indeed from this one side only. I now find that the dream-work is altogether excellently adapted to the peculiarities of wit. This conception is now concluded; if the conclusion leads us not to a familiar province, but rather to one that is strange and novel to our modes of thought, the conclusion is called a "hypothesis," and the relation of the hypothesis to the material from which it is drawn is justly not accepted as "proof." The hypothesis is admitted as "proved" only if it can be reached by other ways and if it can be shown to be the junction point for other associations. But such proof, in view of the fact that our knowledge of unconscious processes has hardly begun, cannot be had. Realizing then that we are on soil still virgin, we shall be content to project from our viewpoint of observation one narrow slender plank into the unexplored region.

We shall not build a great structure on such a foundation as this. If we correlate the different stages of wit to the mental dispositions favorable to them we may say: The *jest* has its origin in the happy mood; what seems to be peculiar to it is an inclination to lower the psychic static energies (*Besetzungen*). The jest already makes use of all the characteristic techniques of wit and satisfies the fundamental conditions of the same through the choice of such an assortment of words or mental associations as will conform not only to the requirements for the production of pleasure, but also conform to the demands of the intelligent critic. We shall conclude that the sinking of the mental energy to the unconscious stage, a process facilitated by the happy mood, has already taken place in the case of the jest. The mood does away with this requirement in the case of *harmless* wit connected with the expression of a valuable thought; here we must assume a particular *personal adaptation* which finds it as easy to come to expression as it is for the foreconscious thought to sink for a moment into the unconscious. An ever watchful tendency to renew the original resultant pleasure of wit exerts thereby a lowering effect upon the still fluctuating foreconscious expression of the thought. Most people are probably capable of making jests when in a happy mood; aptitude for joking independent of the mood is found only in a few persons. Finally, the most powerful incentive for wit-work is the presence of strong tendencies which reach back into the unconscious and which indicate a particular fitness for witty productions; these tendencies might explain to us why the subjective conditions of wit are so frequently fulfilled in the case of neurotic persons. Even the most inapt person may become witty under the influence of strong tendencies.

Differences Between Wit and Dreams

This last contribution, the explanation of wit-work in the first person, though still hypothetical, strictly speaking, ends our interest in wit. There still remains a short comparison of wit to the more familiar dream and we may expect that, outside of the one agreement already considered, two such diverse mental activities should show nothing but differences. The most important difference lies in their social behavior. The dream is a perfectly asocial psychic product. It has nothing to tell to anyone else, having originated in an individual as a compromise between conflicting psychic forces it remains incomprehensible to the person himself and has therefore altogether no interest for anybody else. Not only does the dream find it unnecessary to place any value on intelligibleness, but it must even guard against being understood, as it would then be destroyed; it can only exist in disguised form. For this reason the dream may make use freely of the mechanism that controls unconscious thought processes to the extent of producing undecipherable disfigurements. Wit, on the other hand, is the most social of all those psychic functions whose aim is to gain pleasure. It often requires three persons, and the psychic process which it incites always requires the participation of at least one other person. It must therefore bind itself to the condition of intelligibleness; it may employ disfigurement made practicable in the unconscious through condensation and displacement, to no greater extent than can be deciphered by the intelligence of the third person. As for the rest, wit and dreams have developed in altogether different spheres of the psychic life, and are to be classed under widely separated categories of the psychological system. No matter how concealed the dream is still a wish, while wit is a developed play. Despite its apparent unreality the dream retains its relation to the great interests of life; it seeks to supply what is lacking through a regressive detour of hallucinations; and it owes its existence solely to the strong need for sleep during the night. Wit, on the other hand, seeks to draw a small amount of pleasure from the free and unencumbered activities of our psychic apparatus, and later to seize this pleasure as an incidental gain. It thus *secondarily* reaches to important functions relative to the outer world. The dream serves preponderately to guard from pain while wit serves to acquire pleasure; in these two aims all our psychic activities meet.

VII

WE have approached the problems of the comic in an unusual manner. It appeared to us that wit, which is usually regarded as a subspecies of the comic, offered enough peculiarities to warrant our taking it directly under consideration, and thus it came about that we avoided discussing its relation to the more comprehensive category of the comic as long as it was possible to do so, yet we did not proceed without picking up on the way some hints that might be valuable for studying the comic. We found it easy to ascertain that the comic differs from wit in its social behavior. The comic can be content with only two persons, one who finds the comical, and one in whom it is found. The third person to whom the comical may be imparted reinforces the comic process, but adds nothing new to it. In wit, however, this third person is indispensable for the completion of the pleasure-bearing process, while the second person may be omitted, especially when it is not a question of aggressive wit with a tend-

288

ency. Wit is made, while the comical is found; it is found first of all in persons, and only later by transference may be seen also in objects, situations, and the like. We know, too, in the case of wit that it is not strange persons, but one's own mental processes that contain the sources for the production of pleasure. In addition we have heard that wit occasionally reopens inaccessible sources of the comic, and that the comic often serves wit as a façade to replace the fore-pleasure usually produce by the well-known technique (p. 236). All of this does not really point to a very simple relationship between wit and the comic. On the other hand, the problems of the comic have shown themselves to be so complicated, and have until now so successfully defied all attempts made by the philosophers to solve them, that we have not been able to justify the expectation of mastering it by a sudden stroke, so to speak, even if we approach it along the paths of wit. Incidentally we came provided with an instrument for investigating wit that had not yet been made use of by others; namely, the knowledge of dream-work. We have no similar advantage at our disposal for comprehending the comic, and we may therefore expect that we shall learn nothing about the nature of the comic other than

that which we have already become aware of
in wit; in so far as wit belongs to the comic
and retains certain features of the same unchanged or modified in its own nature.

The Naïve

The species of the comic that is most closely
allied to wit is the *naïve*. Like the comic the
naïve is found universally and is not made like
in the case of wit. The naïve cannot be made
at all, while in the case of the pure comic the
question of making or evoking the comical may
be taken into account. The naïve must result without our intervention from the speech
and actions of other persons who take the place
of the *second* person in the comic or in wit.
The naïve originates when one puts himself
completely outside of inhibition, because it
does not exist for him; that is, if he seems to
overcome it without any effort. What conditions the function of the naïve is the fact that
we are aware that the person does not possess
this inhibition, otherwise we should not call it
naïve but impudent, and instead of laughing
we should be indignant. The effect of the
naïve, which is irresistible, seems easy to understand. An expenditure of that inhibition energy which is commonly already formed in us

suddenly becomes inapplicable when we hear the naïve and is discharged through laughter; as the removal of the inhibition is direct, and not the result of an incited operation, there is no need for a suspension of attention. We behave like the hearer in wit, to whom the economy of inhibition is given without any effort on his part.

In view of the understanding about the genesis of inhibitions which we obtained while tracing the development of play into wit, it will not surprise us to learn that the naïve is mostly found in children, although it may also be observed in uneducated adults, whom we look on as children as far as their intellectual development is concerned. For the purposes of comparison with wit, naïve speech is naturally better adapted than naïve actions, for speech and not actions are the usual forms of expression employed by wit. It is significant, however, that naïve speeches, such as those of children, can without straining also be designated as " naïve witticisms." The points of agreement as well as demonstration between wit and naïveté will become clear to us upon consideration of a few examples.[1]

A little girl of three years was accustomed to hear from her German nurse the exclamatory

[1] Given by Translator.

*word " Gesundheit " (God bless you!; liter-
ally, may you be healthy!) whenever she happened to sneeze. While suffering from a severe cold during which the profuse coughing
and sneezing caused her considerable pain, she
pointed to her chest and said to her father,
" Daddy, Gesundheit hurts."*

*Another little girl of four years heard her
parents refer to a Jewish acquaintance as a
Hebrew, and on later hearing the latter's wife
referred to as Mrs. X, she corrected her
mother, saying, " No, that is not her name; if
her husband is a Hebrew she is a Shebrew."*

In the first example the wit is produced
through the use of a contiguous association in
the form of an abstract thought for the concrete action. The child so often heard the
word " Gesundheit " associated with sneezing
that she took it for the act itself. While the
second example may be designated as word-
wit formed by the technique of sound similarity. The child divided the word Hebrew into
He-brew and having been taught the genders
of the personal pronouns, she naturally
imagined that if the man is a He-brew his wife
must be a She-brew. Both examples could
have originated as real witticisms upon which
we would have unwillingly bestowed a little
mild laughter. But as examples of naïveté

they seem excellent and cause loud laughter. But what is it here that produces the difference between wit and naïveté? Apparently it is neither the wording nor the technique, which is the same for both wit and the naïve, but a factor which at first sight seems remote from both. It is simply a question whether we assume that the speakers had the intention of making a witticism or whether we assume that they—the children—wished to draw an earnest conclusion, a conclusion held in good faith though based on uncorrected knowledge. Only the latter case is one of naïveté. It is here that our attention is first called to the mechanism in which the second person places himself into the psychic process of the person who produces the wit.

The investigation of a third example will confirm this opinion. A brother and a sister, the former ten and the latter twelve years old, produce a play of their own composition before an audience of uncles and aunts. The scene represents a hut on the seashore. In the first act the two dramatist-actors, a poor fisherman and his devoted wife, complain about the hard times and the difficulty of getting a livelihood. The man decides to sail over the wide ocean in his boat in order to seek wealth elsewhere, and after a touching farewell the curtain is drawn. The second act takes place several years later. The fisherman has come home rich with a big bag of money and tells his wife, whom he finds waiting in front of the hut, what good luck he has had in the far countries. His wife interrupts him proudly, saying: " Nor have I been idle in the meanwhile," and opens the hut, on whose floor the fisherman sees twelve large dolls representing children asleep. At this point of the drama the performers were interrupted by an outburst of laughter on the part of the audience, a thing which they could not understand. They stared dumfounded at their dear relatives, who had thus far behaved respectably and had listened attentively. The explanation of this laughter lies in the assumption on the part of the audience that the young dramatists know nothing as yet about the origin of children, and were therefore in a position to believe that a wife would actually boast of bearing offspring during the prolonged absence of her husband, and that the husband would rejoice with her over it. But the results achieved by the dramatists on the basis of this ignorance may be designated as nonsense or absurdity.

These examples show that the naïve occupies a position midway between wit and the comic. As far as wording and contents are concerned, the naïve speech is identical with wit; it produces a misuse of words, a bit of nonsense, or an obscenity. But the psychic process of the first person or producer which, in the case of wit, offered us so much that was interesting and puzzling, is here entirely absent. The naïve person imagines that he is using his thoughts and expressions in a simple and normal manner; he has no other purpose in view, and receives no pleasure from his naïve production. All the characteristics of the naïve lie in the conception of the hearer, who corresponds to the third person in the case of wit. The producing person creates the naïve without any effort. The complicated technique, which in wit serves to paralyze the inhibition produced by the critical reason, does not exist here, because the person does not possess this inhibition, and he can therefore readily produce the senseless and the obscene without any compromise. The naïve may be added to the realm of wit if it comes into existence after the important function of the censor, as observed in the formula for wit-formation, has been reduced to zero.

If the affective determination of wit consists in the fact that both persons should be subject to about the same inhibitions or inner resistances, we may say now that the determination of the naïve consists in the fact that one person should have inhibitions which the other lacks. It is the person provided with inhibitions who understands the naïve, and it is he alone who gains the pleasure produced by the naïve. We can easily understand that this pleasure is due to the removal of inhibitions. Since the pleasure of wit is of the same origin —a kernel of word-pleasure and nonsense-pleasure, and a shell of removal- and release-pleasure,—the similarity of this connection to the inhibition thus determines the inner relationship between the naïve and wit. In both cases pleasure results from the removal of inner inhibitions. But the psychic process of the recipient person (which in the naïve regularly corresponds with our ego, whereas in wit we may also put ourselves in place of the producing person) is by as much more complicated in the case of the naïve as it is simpler in the producing person in wit. For one thing, the naïve must produce the same effect upon the receiving person as wit does, this may be fully confirmed by our examples, for just as in wit the removal of the censor has been made possible by the mere effort of hearing the naïve. But only a part of the pleasure created by the naïve admits of this explanation, in other cases of naïve utterances, even this portion would be endangered, as, for example, while listening to naïve obscenities. We would react to a naïve obscenity with the same indignation felt toward a real obscenity, were it not for the fact that another factor saves us from this indignation and at the same time furnishes the more important part of the pleasure derived from the naïve.

This other factor is the result of the condition mentioned before, namely, that in order to recognize the naïve we have to be cognizant of the fact that there are no inner inhibitions in the producing person. It is only when this is assured that we laugh instead of being indignant. Hence we take into consideration the psychic state of the producing person; we imagine ourselves in this same psychic state and endeavor to understand it by comparing it to our own. This putting ourselves into the psychic state of the producing person and comparing it with our own results in an economy of expenditure which we discharge through laughing.

We might prefer the simpler explanation, namely, that when we reflect that the person has no inhibition to overcome our indignation becomes superfluous; the laughing therefore results at the cost of economized indignation. In order to avoid this conception, which is, in

general, misleading, I shall distinguish more
sharply between two cases that I had treated
as one in the above discussion. The naïve, as
it appears to us, may either be in the nature
of a witticism, as in our example, or an obscenity, or of anything generally objectionable;
which becomes especially evident if the naïve
is expressed not in speech but in action.
This latter case is really misleading; for
it might lead one to assume that the pleasure originated from the economized and transformed indignation. The first case is the il-
luminating one. The naïve speech in the example "Hebrew" can produce the effect of a
light witticism and give no cause for indignation; it is certainly the more rare, or the more
pure and by far the more instructive case. In
so far as we think that the child took the syllable "he" in "Hebrew" seriously, and without
any additional reason identified it with the
masculine personal pronoun, the increase in
pleasure as a result of hearing it has no longer
anything to do with the pleasure of the wit.
We shall now consider what has been said
from two viewpoints, first how it came into
existence in the mind of the child, and secondly, how it would occur to us. In following this comparison we find that the child has
discovered an identity and has overcome bar-

riers which exist in us, and by continuing still further it may express itself as follows: " If you wish to understand what you have heard, you may save yourself the expenditure necessary for holding these barriers in place." The expenditure which became freed by this comparison is the source of pleasure in the naïve, and is discharged through laughter; to be sure, it is the same expenditure which we would have converted into indignation if our understanding of the producing person, and in this case the nature of his utterance, had not precluded it. But if we take the case of the naïve joke as a model for the second case, viz., the objectionable naïve, we shall see that here, too, the economy in inhibition may originate directly from the comparison. That is, it is unnecessary for us to assume an incipient and then a strangulated indignation, an indignation corresponding to a different application of the freed expenditure, against which, in the case of wit, complicated defensive mechanisms were required.

Source of Comic Pleasure in the Naïve

This comparison and this economy of expenditure that occur as the result of putting one's self into the psychic process of the producing person can have an important bearing on the naïve only if they do not belong to the naïve alone. As a matter of fact we suspect that this mechanism which is so completely foreign to wit is a part—perhaps the essential part—of the psychic process of the comic. This aspect—it is perhaps the most important aspect of the naïve—thus represents the naïve as a form of the comic. Whatever is added to the wit-pleasure by the naïve speeches in our examples is "comical" pleasure. Concerning the latter we might be inclined to make a general assumption that this pleasure originates through an economized expenditure by comparing the utterance of some one else with our own. But since we are here in the presence of very broad views we shall first conclude our consideration of the naïve. The naïve would thus be a form of the comic, in so far as its pleasure originates from the difference in expenditure which results in our effort to understand the other person; and it resembles wit through the condition that the expenditure saved by the comparison must be an inhibition expenditure.[1]

---

[1] I have everywhere identified the naïve with the naïve-comic, a practice which is certainly not permissible in all cases. But it is sufficient for our purposes to study the characteristics of the naïve as exhibited by the "naïve joke" and the "naïve obscenity." It is our intention to proceed from here with the investigation of the nature of the comic.

Before concluding we shall rapidly point out a few agreements and differences between the conceptions at which we have just arrived and those that have been known for a long time in the psychology of the comic. The putting one's self into the psychic process of another and the desire to understand him is obviously nothing else than the "comic burrowing" (*komisches Leihen*) which has played a part in the analysis of the comic ever since the time of Jean Paul; the "comparing" of the psychic process of another with our own corresponds to a "psychological contrast," for which we here at last find a place, after we did not know what to do with it in wit. But in our explanation of comic pleasure we take issue with many authors who contend that this pleasure originates through the fluctuation of our attention to and fro between contrasting ideas. We are unable to see how such a mechanism could produce pleasure, and we point to the fact that in the comparing of contrasts there results a difference in expenditure which, if not used for anything else, becomes capable of discharge and hence a source of pleasure.[1]

[1] Also Bergson (*Laughter*, An essay on the Meaning of the Comic, translated by Brereton and Rothwell, The Macmillan Co., 1914) rejects with sound arguments this sort of explanation of comic pleasure, which has unmistakably been influenced by the effort to create an analogy to the laughing of a person tickled.

It is with misgiving only that we approach the problem of the comic. It would be presumptuous to expect from our efforts any decisive contribution to the solution of this problem after the works of a large number of excellent thinkers have not resulted in an explanation that is in every respect satisfactory. As a matter of fact, we intend simply to follow out into the province of the comic certain observations that have been found valuable in the study of wit.

Occurrence and Origin of the Comic

The comical appears primarily as an unintentional discovery in the social relations of human beings. It is found in persons, that is, in their movements, shapes, actions, and characteristic traits. In the beginning it is found probably only in their psychical peculiarities and later on in their mental qualities, especially in the expression of these latter. Even animals and inanimate objects become comical as the result of a widely used method of personification. However, the comical can be considered apart from the person in whom it is found, if the conditions under which a person becomes

The explanation of comic pleasure by Lipps which might, in connection with his conception of the comic, be represented as an "unexpected trifle," is of an entirely different nature.

comical can be discerned. Thus arises the comical situation, and this knowledge enables us to make a person comical at will by putting him into situations in which the conditions necessary for the comic are bound up with his actions. The discovery that it is in our power to make another person comical opens the way to unsuspected gains in comic pleasure, and forms the foundation of a highly developed technique. It is also possible to make one's self just as comical as others. The means which serve to make a person comical are transference into comic situations, imitations, disguise, unmasking, caricature, parody travesty, and the like. It is quite evident that these techniques may enter into the service of hostile or aggressive tendencies. A person may be made comical in order to render him contemptible or in order to deprive him of his claims to dignity and authority. But even if such a purpose were regularly at the bottom of all attempts to make a person comical this need not necessarily be the meaning of the spontaneous comic.

As a result of this superficial survey of the manifestations of the comic we can readily see that the comic originates from wide-spread sources, and that conditions so specialized as those found in the naïve cannot be expected in the case of the comic. In order to get a clue to the conditions that are applicable to the comic the selection of the first example is most important. We will examine first the comic movement because we remember that the most primitive stage performance, the pantomime, uses this means to make us laugh. The answer to the question, Why do we laugh at the actions of clowns? would be that they appear to us immoderate and inappropriate; that is, we really laugh over the excessive expenditure of energy. Let us look for the same condition outside of the manufactured comic, that is, under circumstances where it may unintentionally be found. The child's motions do not appear to us comical, even if it jumps and fidgets, but it is comical to see a little boy or girl follow with the tongue the movement of his pen-holder when he is trying to master the art of writing; we see in these additional motions a superfluous expenditure of energy which under similar conditions we should save. In the same way we find it comical to see unnecessary motions or even marked exaggeration of expressive motions in adults. Among the genuinely comic cases we might mention the motions made by the bowler after he has released the ball while he is following its course as though he were still able to control it; all grimaces which exaggerate the normal expression of the emotions are comical, even if they are involuntary, as in the case of persons suffering from St. Vitus' dance (chorea); the impassioned movements of a modern orchestra leader will appear comical to every unmusical person, who cannot understand why they are necessary. Indeed, the comic element found in bodily shapes and physiognomy is a branch of the comic of motion, in that they are conceived as though they were the result of motion that either has been carried too far or is purposeless. Wide exposed eyes, a crook-shaped nose bent towards the mouth, handle-like ears, a hunch back, and all similar physical defects probably produce a comical impression only in so far as the movements that would be necessary to produce these features are imagined, whereby the nose and other parts of the body are pictured as more movable than they actually are. It is certainly comical if some one can " wiggle his ears," and it would undoubtedly be a great deal more comical if he could raise and lower his nose. A large part of the comical impression that animals make upon us is due to the fact that we perceive in them movements which we cannot imitate.

Comic of Motion

But how does it come about that we laugh as soon as we have recognized that the actions of some one else are immoderate and inappropriate? I believe that we laugh because we compare the motions observed in others with those which we ourselves should produce if we were in their place. The two persons must naturally be compared in accordance with the same standard, but this standard is my own innervation expenditure connected with my idea of motion in the one case as well as the other. This assertion is in need of discussion and amplification.

What we are here putting into juxtaposition is, on the one hand, the psychic expenditure of a given idea, and on the other hand, the content of this idea. We maintain that the former is not primarily and principally independent of the latter—the content of the idea—particularly because the idea of something great requires a larger expenditure than the idea of something small. As long as we are concerned only with the idea of different coarse movements we shall encounter no difficulties in the theoretical determination of our thesis or in establishing its proof through observation. It will be shown that in this case

an attribute of the idea actually coincides with
an attribute of the object conceived, although
psychology warns us of confusions of this sort.

I obtain an idea of a definite coarse movement by performing this motion or by imitating it, and in so doing I set a standard for
this motion in my feelings of innervation.[1]

Now if I perceive a similar more or less
coarse motion in some one else, the surest way
to the understanding—to apperception—of the
same is to carry it out imitatively and the comparison will then enable me to decide in which
motion I expended more energy. Such an impulse to imitate certainly arises on perceiving
a movement. But in reality I do not carry
out the imitation any more than I still spell
out words simply because I have learnt to read
by means of spelling. Instead of imitating the
movement by my muscles I substitute the idea
of the same through my memory traces of the
expenditures necessary for similar motions.
Perceiving, or "thinking," differs above all

[1] The recollection of this innervation expenditure will remain
the essential part of the idea of this motion, and there will
always be methods of thought in my psychic life in which the
idea will be represented by nothing else than this expenditure.
In other connections a substitute for this element may possibly
be put in the form of other ideas, for instance the visual idea
of the object of the motion, or it may be put in the form of the
word-idea; and in certain types of abstract thought a sign instead of the full content itself may suffice.

from acting or carrying out things by the fact that it entails a very much smaller displacement of energy and keeps the main expenditure from being discharged. But how is the quantitative factor, the more or less big element of the movement perceived, given expression in the idea? And if the representation of the quantity is left off from the idea that is composed of qualities, how am I to differentiate the ideas of different big movements, how am I to compare them?

Here, physiology shows the way in that it teaches us that even while an idea is in the process of conception innervations proceed to the muscles, which naturally represent only a moderate expenditure. It is now easy to assume that this expenditure of innervation which accompanies the conception of the idea is utilized to represent the quantitative factor of the idea, and that when a great motion is imagined it is greater than it would be in the case of a small one. The conception of greater motions would thus actually be greater, that is, it would be a conception accompanied by greater expenditure.

Ideational Mimicry

Observation shows directly that human beings are in the habit of expressing the big and small things in their ideation content by means of a manifold expenditure or by means of a sort of *ideational mimicry.*

When a child or a person of the common people or one belonging to a certain race imparts or depicts something, one can easily observe that he is not content to make his ideas intelligible to the hearer through the choice of correct words alone, but that he also represents the contents of the same through his expressive motions. Thus he designates the quantities and intensities of " a high mountain " by raising his hands over his head, and those of " a little dwarf " by lowering his hand to the ground. If he broke himself of the habit of depicting with his hands, he would nevertheless do it with his voice, and if he should also control his voice, one may be sure that in picturing something big he would distend his eyes, and describing something little he would press his eyes together. It is not his own affects that he thus expresses, but it is really the content of what he imagines.

Shall we now assume that this need for mimicry is first aroused through the demand for imparting, whereas a good part of this manner of representation still escapes the attention of the hearer? I rather believe that this mimicry, though less vivid, exists even if all

imparting is left out of the question, that it
comes about when the person imagines for
himself alone, or thinks of something in a
graphic manner; that then such a person, just
as in talking, expresses through his body the
idea of big and small which manifests itself at
least through a change of innervation in the
facial expressions and sensory organs. Indeed,
I can imagine that the bodily innervation
which is consensual to the content of the idea
conceived is the beginning and origin of mimicry for purposes of communication. For, in
order to be in a position to serve this purpose,
it is only necessary to increase it and make it
conspicuous to the other. When I take the
view that this "expression of the ideation content" should be added to the expression of the
emotions, which are known as a physical by-
effect of psychic processes, I am well aware
that my observations which refer to the category of the big and small do not exhaust
the subject. I myself could add still other
things, even before reaching to the phenomenon of tension through which a person
physically indicates the accumulation of his attention and the *niveau* of abstraction upon
which his thoughts happen to rest. I maintain
that this subject is very important, and I believe that tracing the ideation mimicry in other

fields of æsthetics would be just as useful for the understanding of the comic as it is here.

To return to the comic movement, I repeat that with the perception of a certain motion the impulse to conceive it will be given through a certain expenditure. In the "desire to understand," in the apperception of this movement I produce a certain expenditure, and I behave in this part of the psychic process just as if I put myself in the place of the person observed. Simultaneously I probably grasp the aim of the motion, and through former experiences I am able to estimate the amount of expenditure necessary to attain this aim. I thereby drop out of consideration the person observed and behave as if I myself wished to attain the aim of the motion. These two ideational possibilities depend on a comparison of the motion observed with my own inhibited motion. In the case of an immoderate or inappropriate movement on the part of the other, my greater expenditure for understanding becomes inhibited *statu nascendi* during the mobilization as it were, it is declared superfluous and stands free for further use or for discharge through laughing. If other favorable conditions supervened this would be the nature of the origin of pleasure in comic movement,—an innervation expenditure which,

when compared with one's own motion, becomes an inapplicable surplus.

Comparison of Two Kinds of Expenditure as Pleasure-sources

We now note that we must continue our
discussion by following two different paths;
first, to determine the conditions for the discharge of the surplus; secondly, to test
whether the other cases of the comic can be
conceived similarly to our conception of comic
motion.

We shall turn first to the latter task and
after considering comic movement and action
we shall turn to the comic found in the psychic activities and peculiarities of others.

As an example of this kind we may consider the comical nonsense produced by ignorant students at examinations; it is more difficult, however, to give a simple example of
the peculiarities. We must not be confused
by the fact that nonsense and foolishness which
so often act in a comical manner are nevertheless not perceived as comical in all cases, just
as the same things which once made us laugh
because they seemed comical later may appear
to us contemptible and hateful. This fact,
which we must not forget to take into account,

seems only to show that besides the comparison familiar to us other relations come into consideration for the comic effect,—conditions which we can investigate in other connections.

The comic found in the mental and psychic attributes of another person is apparently again the result of a comparison between him and my own ego. But it is remarkable that it is a comparison which mostly furnishes the result opposite to that obtained through comic movement and action. In the latter case it is comical if the other person assumes a greater expenditure than I believe to be necessary for me; in the case of psychic activity it is just the reverse, it is comical if the other person economizes in expenditure, which I consider indispensable; for nonsense and foolishness are nothing but inferior activities. In the first case I laugh because he makes it too difficult for himself, and in the latter case because he makes it too easy for himself. In the case of the comic effect it seems to be a question only of the difference between the two energy expenditures—the one of " feeling one's self into something" (*Einfühlung*)—and the other of the ego—and it makes no difference in whose favor this difference inclines. This peculiarity, which at first confuses our judgment, disappears, however, when we consider that it is in

accord with our personal development towards
a higher stage of culture, to limit our muscular
work and increase our mental work. By
heightening our mental expenditure we produce a diminution of motion expenditure for
the same activity. Our machines bear witness
to this cultural success.[1]

Thus it coincides with a uniform understanding that that person appears comical to us who
puts forth too much expenditure in his psychical
activities and too little in his mental activities;
and it cannot be denied that in both cases our
laughing is the expression of a pleasurably
perceived superiority which we adjudge to
ourselves in comparison with him. If the relation in both cases becomes reversed, that is,
if the somatic expenditure of the other is less
and the psychic expenditure greater, then we
no longer laugh, but are struck with amaze-
ment and admiration.[2]

Comic of Situation.

The origin of the comic pleasure discussed here,
that is, the origin of such pleasure in a com-

[1] "What one has not in his head," as the saying goes, "he
must have in his legs."

[2] The problem has been greatly confused by the general conditions determining the comic, whereby the comic pleasure is seen
to have its source now in a too-muchness and now in a not-
enoughness.

parison of the other person with one's own self
in respect to the difference between the identification expenditure (*Einfühlungsaufwand*)
and normal expenditure—is genetically probably the most important. It is certain, however,
that it is not the only one. We have learned
before to disregard any such comparison between the other person and one's self, and to
obtain the pleasure-bringing difference from
one side only, either from identification, or
from the processes in one's own ego, proving
thereby that the feeling of superiority bears
no essential relations to comic pleasure. A
comparison is indispensable, however, for the
origin of this pleasure, and we find this comparison between two energy expenditures
which rapidly follow each other and refer to
the same function. It is produced either in
ourselves by way of identification with the
other, or we find it without any identification
in our own psychic processes. The first case,
in which the other person still plays a part,
though he is not compared with ourselves, results when the pleasure-producing difference
of energy expenditures comes into existence
through outer influences which we can comprehend as a "situation," for which reason this
species of comic is also called the "comic of
situation." The peculiarities of the person who

furnishes the comic do not here come into essential consideration; we laugh when we admit
to ourselves that had we been placed in the
same situation we should have done the same
thing. Here we draw the comic from the relation of the individual to the often all-too-
powerful outer world, which is represented in
the psychic processes of the individual by the
conventions and necessities of society, and even
by his bodily needs. A typical example of the
latter is when a person engaged in an activity,
which claims all his psychic forces, is suddenly
disturbed by a pain or excremental need. The
opposite case which furnishes us the comic
difference through identification, lies between
the great interest which existed before the
disturbance occurred and the minimum left
for his psychic activity after the disturbance made its appearance. The person who
furnishes us this difference again becomes
comical through inferiority; but he is only inferior in comparison with his former ego and
not in comparison with us, for we know that
in a similar case we could not have behaved
differently. It is remarkable, however, that
we find this inferiority of the person only in
the case where we " feel ourselves " into some
one, that is, we can only find it comical in the
other, whereas we ourselves are conscious only

of painful emotions when such or similar embarrassments happen to us. It is by keeping away the painful from our own person that we are probably first enabled to enjoy as pleasurable the difference which resulted from the comparison of the changing energy.

Comic of Expectation

The other source of the comic, which we find in our own changes of investing energy, lies in our relations to the future, which we are accustomed to anticipate through our ideas of expectation. I assume that a quantitatively determined expenditure underlies our every idea of expectation, which in case of disappointment becomes diminished by a certain difference, and I again refer to the observations made before concerning "ideational mimicry." But it seems to me easier to demonstrate the real mobilized psychic expenditure for the cases of expectation. It is well known concerning a whole series of cases that the manifestation of expectation is formed by motor preliminaries; this is first of all true of cases in which the expected events make demands on my motility, and these preparations are quantitatively determinable without anything further. If I am expecting to catch a ball

thrown at me, I put my body in states of tension in order to enable me to withstand the
collision with the ball, and the superfluous motions which I make if the ball turns out to be
light make me look comical to the spectators.
I allowed myself to be misled by the expectation to exert an immoderate expenditure of
motion. A similar thing happens if, for example, I lift out a basket of fruit which I took
to be heavy but which was hollow and formed
out of wax in order to deceive me. By its up-
ward jerk my arm betrays the fact that I have
prepared a superfluous innervation for this
purpose and hence I am laughed at. In fact
there is at least one case in which the expectation expenditure can be directly demonstrated
by means of physiological experimentation with
animals. In Pawlof's experiments with sali-
vary secretions of dogs who, provided with sali-
vary fistulæ, are shown different kinds of food,
it is noticed that the amount of saliva secreted
through the fistulæ depends on whether the
conditions of the experiment have strengthened
or disappointed the dogs' expectation to be
fed with the food shown them.

Even where the thing expected lays claims
only to my sensory organs, and not to my motility, I may assume that the expectation manifests itself in a certain motor emanation caus-

ing tension of the senses, and I may even conceive the suspension of attention as a motor activity which is equivalent to a certain amount of expenditure. Moreover, I can presuppose that the preparatory activity of expectation is not independent of the amount of the expected impression, but that I represent mimically the bigness and smallness of the same by means of a greater or smaller preparatory expenditure, just as in the case of imparting something and in the case of thinking when there is no expectation. The expectation expenditure naturally will be composed of many components, and also for my disappointment diverse factors will come into consideration; it is not only a question whether the realized event is perceptibly greater or smaller than the expected one, but also whether the expectation is worthy of the great interest which I had offered for it. In this manner I am instructed to consider, besides the expenditure for the representation of bigness and smallness (the conceptual mimicry), also the expenditure for the tension of attention (expectation expenditure), and in addition to these two expenditures there is in all cases the abstraction expenditure. But these other forms of expenditure can easily be reduced to the one of bigness and smallness, for what we call more interesting, more sublime, and even more abstract, are only particularly qualified special cases of what is greater. Let us add to this that, among other things, Lipps holds that the quantitative, not the qualitative, contrast is primarily the source of comic pleasure and we shall be altogether content to have chosen the comic element of motion as the starting-point of our investigation.

In working out Kant's thesis, "The comic is an expectation dwindled into nothing," Lipps made the attempt in his book, often cited here, to trace the comic pleasure altogether to expectation. Despite the many instructive and valuable results which this attempt brought to light I should like to agree with the criticism expressed by other authors, namely, that Lipps has formulated a field of origin of the comic which is much too narrow, and that he could not subject its phenomena to his formula without much forcing.

Caricature

Human beings are not satisfied with enjoying the comic as they encounter it in life, but they aim to produce it purposely, thus we discover more of the nature of the comic by studying the methods employed in producing the comic. Above all one can produce comical elements in one's personality for the amusement of others, by making one's self appear awkward or stupid. One then produces the comic exactly as if one were really so, by complying with the condition of comparison which leads to the difference of expenditure; but one does not make himself laughable or contemptible through this; indeed, under certain circumstances one can even secure admiration. The feeling of superiority does not come into existence in the other when he knows that the actor is only shamming, and this furnishes us a good new proof that the comic is independent in principle of the feeling of superiority.

To make another comical, the method most commonly employed is to transfer him into situations wherein he becomes comical regardless of his personal qualities, as a result of human dependence upon external circumstances, especially social factors; in other words, one resorts to the comical situation. This transferring into a comic situation may be real as in practical jokes, such as placing the foot in front of one so that he falls like a clumsy person, or making one appear stupid by utilizing his credulity to make him believe some nonsense, etc., or it can be feigned by means of speech or play. It is a good aid in aggression, in the service of which production of the comic is wont to place itself in order that the comic pleasure may be independent of the reality of the comic situation; thus every person is really defenseless against being made comical.

But there are still other means of making one comical which deserve special attention and which in part also show new sources of comic pleasure. *Imitation,* for example, belongs here; it accords the hearer an extraordinary amount of pleasure and makes its subject comic, even if it still keeps away from the exaggeration of caricature. It is much easier to fathom the comic effect of caricature than that of simple imitation. Caricature, parody and travesty like their practical counterpart—unmasking, range themselves against persons and objects who command authority and respect and who are exalted in some sense—these are procedures tending towards degradation.[1] In the transferred psychic sense, the exalted is equivalent to something great and I want to make the statement, or more accurately to repeat the statement, that psychic greatness like somatic greatness

---

[1] Degradation: A. Bain (*The Emotions and the Will,* 2nd Ed., 1865) states: "The occasion of the ludicrous is the degradation of some person of interest possessing dignity, in circumstances that excite no other strong emotion" (p. 248).

is exhibited by means of an increased expenditure. It needs little observation to ascertain that when I speak of the exalted I give a different innervation to my voice, I change my facial expression, an attempt to bring my entire bearing as it were into complete accord with the dignity of that which I present. I impose upon myself a dignified restriction not much different than if I were coming into the presence of an illustrious personage, monarch, or prince of science. I can scarcely err when I assume that this added innervation of conceptual mimicry corresponds to an increased expenditure. The third case of such an added expenditure I readily find when I indulge in abstract trains of thought instead of in the concrete and plastic ideas. If I can now imagine that the mentioned processes for degrading the illustrious are quite ordinary, that during their activity I need not be on my guard and in whose ideal presence I may, to use a military formula, put myself " at ease," all that saves me the added expenditure of dignified restriction. Moreover, the comparison of this manner of presentation instigated by identification with the manner of presentation to which I have been hitherto accustomed which seeks to present itself at the same time, again produces a difference in expenditure which can be discharged through laughter.

As is known, caricature brings about the degradation by rendering prominent one feature, comic in itself, from the entire picture of the exalted object, a feature which would be overlooked if viewed with the entire picture. Only by isolating this feature can the comic effect be obtained which spreads in our memory over the whole picture. This has, however, this condition; the presence of the exalted itself must not force us into a disposition of reverence. Where such a comical feature is really lacking then caricature unhesitatingly creates it by exaggerating one that is not comical in itself. It is again characteristic of the origin of comic pleasure that the effect of the caricature is not essentially impaired through such a falsifying of reality.

Unmasking

Parody and *travesty* accomplish the degradation of the exalted by other means; they destroy the uniformity between the attributes of persons familiar to us and their speech and actions; by replacing either the illustrious persons or their utterances by lowly ones. Therein they differ from caricature, but not

through the mechanism of the production of
the comic pleasure. The same mechanism also
holds true in *unmasking*, which comes into
consideration only where some one has attached
to himself dignity and authority which in
reality should be taken from him. We have
seen the comic effect of unmasking through
several examples of wit, for example, in the
story of the fashionable lady who in her first
labor-pains cries: "Ah, mon Dieu!" but to
whom the physician paid no attention until she
screamed: " A-a-a-ai-e-e-e-e-e-e-E-E-E!" Being now acquainted with the character of the
comic, we can no longer dispute that this story
is really an example of comical unmasking and
has no just claim to the term witticism. It
recalls wit only through the setting, through
the technical means of "representation through
a trifle"; here it is the cry which was found
sufficient to indicate the point. The fact remains, however, that our feeling for the nice-
ties of speech, when we call on it for judgment, does not oppose calling such a story a
witticism. We can find the explanation for
this in the reflection that usage of speech does
not enter scientifically into the nature of wit
so far as we have evolved it by means of this
painstaking examination. As it is a function
of the activities of wit to reopen hidden

sources of comic pleasure (p. 150), every artifice which does not bring to light barefaced
comic may in looser analogy be called a witticism. This is especially true in the case of
unmasking, though in other methods of comic-
making the appellation also holds good.[1]

In the mechanism of "unmasking" one can
also utilize those processes of comic-making
already known to us which degrade the dignity
of individuals in that they call attention to one
of the common human frailties, but particularly to the dependence of his mental functions upon physical needs. Unmasking them
becomes equivalent to the reminder: This or
that one who is admired like a demigod is
only a human being like you and me after all.
Moreover, all efforts in this mechanism serve
to lay bare the monotonous psychic automatism
which is behind wealth and apparent freedom
of psychic achievements. We have become
acquainted with examples of such "unmasking" through the witticisms dealing with marriage agents, and at that time to be sure we
felt doubt whether we could rightly count
these stories as wit. Now we can decide with
more certainty that the anecdote of the echo
who reinforces all assertions of the marriage

[1] "Thus every conscious and clever evocation of the comic is
called wit, be it the comic of views or situations. Naturally we
cannot use this view of wit here." Lipps, l. c., p. 78.

agent and in the end reinforces the latter's admission that the bride has a hunch back with the exclamation " And what a hunch! " is essentially a comic story, an example of the unmasking of the psychic automatism. But here the comic story serves only as a façade; to any one who wishes to note the hidden meaning of the marriage agent, the whole remains a splendidly put together piece of wit. He who does not penetrate so far sees only the comic story. The same is true of the other witticism of the agent who, to refute an objection, finally confirms the truth through the exclamation: " But who in the world would lend them anything? " This is a comic unmasking which serves as a façade for a witticism. Still the character of the wit is here quite evident, as the speech of the agent is at the same time an expression through the opposite. In trying to prove that the people are rich he proves at the same time that they are not rich but very poor. Wit and the comic unite here and teach us that a statement may be simultaneously witty and comical.

We eagerly grasp the opportunity to return from the comic of unmasking to wit, for our real task is to explain the relation between wit and comic and not to determine the nature of the comic. Hence to the case of uncovering the psychic automatism, wherein our feeling left us in doubt as to whether the matter was comical or witty, we add another, the case of nonsense-wit, wherein likewise wit and the comic fuse. But our investigation will ultimately show us that in this second case the meeting of wit and comic may be theoretically deduced.

In the discussion of the techniques of wit we have found that giving free play. to such modes of thinking as are common in the unconscious and which in consciousness are conceived only as " faulty thinking," furnishes the technical means of a great many witticisms. We had then doubted their witty character and were inclined to classify them simply as comic stories. We could come to no decision regarding our uncertainty because in the first place the real character of wit was not familiar to us. Later we found this character by following the analogy to the dream-work as to the compromise formed by the wit-work between the demands of the rational critic and the impulse not to abandon the old word-pleasure and nonsense-pleasure. What thus came into existence as a compromise, when the foreconscious thought was left for a moment to unconscious elaboration, satisfied both demands in all cases, but it presented itself to the critic, in various forms and had to stand various criticisms from it. In one case wit succeeded in surreptitiously assuming the form of an unimportant but none the less admissible proposition; a second time it smuggled itself into the expression of a valuable thought. But within the outer limit of the compromise activity it made no effort to satisfy the critic, and defiantly utilizing the pleasure-sources at its disposal, it appeared before the critic as pure nonsense. It had no fear of provoking contradiction because it could rely on the fact that the hearer would decipher the disfigurement of the expression through the operation of his unconscious and thus give back to it its meaning.

Now in what case will wit appear to the critic as nonsense? Particularly when it makes use of those modes of thought, which are common in the unconscious, but forbidden in conscious thought; that is, when it resorts to faulty thinking. Some of the modes of thinking, of the unconscious, have also been retained in conscious thinking, for example, many forms of indirect expression, allusions, etc., even though their conscious use has to be much restricted. Using these techniques wit will arouse little or no opposition on the part of the critic; but this only happens when it also uses that technical means

with which conscious thought no longer cares
to have anything to do. Wit can still further
avoid offending if it disguises the faulty think-
in by investing it with a semblance of logic
as in the story of the fancy cake and liqueur,
salmon with mayonnaise, and similar ones.
But should it present the faulty thinking un-
disguised, the critic is sure to protest.

The Meeting of Wit and the Comic

In this case, something else comes to the aid
of wit. The faulty thinking, which as a form
of thinking of the unconscious, wit utilizes for
its technique, appears comical to the critic,
although this is not necessarily the case. The
conscious giving of free play to the unconscious
and to those forms of thinking which are rejected as faulty, furnishes a means for the production of comic pleasure. This can be easily
understood, as a greater expenditure is surely
needed for the production of the foreconscious
investing energy than for the giving of free
play to the unconscious. When we hear the
thought which is formed like one from the unconscious we compare it to its correct form,
and this results in a difference of expenditure
which gives origin to comic pleasure. A witticism which makes use of such faulty thinking
as its technique and therefore appears absurd

can produce a comic impression at the same time. If we do not strike the trail of the wit, there remains to us only the comic or funny story.

The story of the borrowed kettle, which showed a hole on being returned, whereupon the borrower excused himself by stating that in the first place he had not borrowed the kettle; secondly, that it already had a hole when he borrowed it; and thirdly, that he had returned it intact without any hole (p. 82), is an excellent example of a purely comic effect through giving free play to one's unconscious modes of thinking. Just this mutual neutralization of several thoughts, each of which is well motivated in itself, is the province of the unconscious. Corresponding to this, the dream in which the unconscious thoughts become manifest, also shows an absence of either—or.[1] These are expressed by putting the thoughts next to one another. In that dream example given in my *Interpretation of Dreams*,[2] which in spite of its complication I have chosen as a type of the work of interpretation, I seek to rid myself of the reproach that I have not removed the pains of a patient by psychic treatment. My arguments are: 1. she is her-

---

[1] At the most this is inserted by the dreamer as an explanation.
[2] l. c., p. 294.

self to blame for her illness, because she does not wish to accept my solution, 2. her pains are of organic origin, therefore none of my concern, 3. her pains are connected with her widowhood, for which I am certainly not to blame, 4. her pains resulted from an injection with a dirty syringe, which was given by another. All these motives follow one another just as though one did not exclude the other. In order to escape the reproach that it was nonsense I had to insert the words "either—or" instead of the "and" of the dream.

A similar comical story is the one which tells of a blacksmith in a Hungarian village who has committed a crime punishable by death; the bürgomaster, however, decreed that not the smith but a tailor was to be hanged, as there were two tailors in the village but only one blacksmith, and the crime had to be expiated. Such a displacement of guilt from one person to another naturally contradicts all laws of conscious logic, but in no ways the mental trends of the unconscious. I am in doubt whether to call this story comic, and still I put the story of the kettle among the witticisms. Now I admit that it is far more correct to designate the latter as comic rather than witty. But now I understand how it happens that my feelings, usually so reliable, can leave me in the lurch as to whether this story be comic or witty. The case in which I cannot come to a conclusion through my feelings is the one in which the comic results through the uncovering of modes of thought which exclusively belong to the unconscious. A story of that kind can be comic and witty at the same time; but it will impress me as being witty even if it be only comic, because the use of the faulty thinking of the unconscious reminds me of wit, just as in the case of the arrangements for the uncovering of the hidden comic discussed before (p. 325).

I must lay great stress upon making clear this most delicate point of my analysis, namely, the relation of wit to the comic, and will therefore supplement what has been said with some negative statements. First of all, I call attention to the fact that the case of the meeting of wit and comic treated here (p. 327) is not identical with the preceding one. I grant it is a fine distinction, but it can be drawn with certainty. In the preceding case the comic originated from the uncovering of the psychic automatism. This is in no way peculiar to the unconscious alone and it does not at all play a conspicuous part in the technique of wit. Unmasking appears only accidentally in relation with wit, in that it serves another technique of wit, namely, representation through the opposite. But in the case of giving free play to unconscious ways of thinking the union of wit and comic is an essential one, because the same method which is used by the first person in wit as the technique of releasing pleasure will naturally produce comic pleasure in the third person.

We might be tempted to generalize this last case and seek the relation of wit to the comic in the fact that the effect of wit upon the third person follows the mechanism of comic pleasure. But there is no question about that; contact with the comic is not in any way found in all nor even in most witticisms; in most cases wit and the comic can be cleanly separated. As often as wit succeeds in escaping the appearance of absurdity, which is to say in most witticisms of double meaning or of allusion, one cannot discover any effect in the hearer resembling the comic. One can make the test with examples previously cited or with some new ones given here.

Congratulatory telegram to be sent to a gambler on his 70th birthday.

" *Trente et quarante* "[1] (word-division with allusion).

---

[1] " Trente et quarante " is a gambling game.

Madame de *Maintenon* was called Madame de *Maintenant* (modification of a name).

We might further believe that at least all jokes with nonsense façades appear comical and must impress us as such. But I recall here the fact that such witticisms often have a different effect on the hearer, calling forth confusion and a tendency to rejection (see foot- note, p. 212). Therefore it evidently depends whether the nonsense of the wit appears comical or common plain nonsense, and the conditions for this we have not yet investigated. Accord- ingly we hold to the conclusion that wit, judg- ing by its nature, can be separated from the comic, and that it unites with it on the one hand only in certain special cases, on the other in the tendency to gain pleasure from intel- lectual sources.

In the course of these examinations con- cerning the relations of wit and the comic there revealed itself to us that distinction which we must emphasize as most significant, and which at the same time points to a psychologically important characteristic of the comic. We had to transfer to the unconscious the source of wit-pleasure; there is no occasion which can be discovered for the same localization of the comic. On the contrary all analyses which we have made thus far indicate that the source of comic pleasure lies in the comparison of two expenditures, both of which we must adjudged to the foreconscious. Wit and the comic can above all be differentiated in the psychic localization; *wit is, so to speak, the contribution to the comic from the sphere of the unconscious.*

Comic of Imitation

We need not blame ourselves for digressing from the subject, for the relation of wit to the comic is really the occasion which urged us to the examination of the comic. But it is time for us to return to the point under discussion, to the treatment of the means which serve to produce the comic. We have advanced the discussion of caricature and unmasking, because from both of them we can borrow several points of similarity for the analysis of the comic of *imitation*. Imitation is mostly replaced by caricature, which consists in the exaggeration of certain otherwise not striking traits, and also bears the character of degradation. Still this does not seem to exhaust the nature of imitation; it is incontestable that in itself it represents an extraordinarily rich source of comic pleasure, for we laugh particularly over faithful imitations. It is not easy to give a satisfactory explanation of this if we do not accept Bergson's view,[1] according to which the comic of imitation is put next to the comic produced by uncovering the psychic automatism. Bergson believes that everything gives a comic impression which manifests itself in the shape of a machine-like inanimate movement in the human being. His law is that "the attitudes, gestures, and movements of the human body are laughable in exact proportion as that body reminds us of a mere machine." He explains the comic of imitation by connecting it with a problem formulated by Pascal in his *Thoughts,* why is it that we laugh at the comparison of two faces that are alike although neither of them excites laughter by itself. "The truth is that a really living life should never repeat itself. Wherever there is repetition or complete similarity, we always suspect some mechanism at work behind the living." Analyze the impression you get from two faces that are too much alike, and you will find that you are thinking of two copies cast in the same mould, or two impressions of the same soul, or two reproductions of the same negative,—in a word, of some manufacturing process or other. This deflection of life towards the mechanical is here the real

[1] Bergson, l. c., p. 29.

cause of laughter (l. c., p. 34). We might say, it is the degradation of the human to the mechanical or inanimate. If we accept these winning arguments of Bergson, it is moreover not difficult to subject his view to our own formula. Taught by experience that every living being is different and demands a definite amount of expenditure from our understanding, we find ourselves disappointed when, as a result of a perfect agreement or deceptive imitation, we need no new expenditure. But we are disappointed in the sense of being relieved, and the expenditure of expectation which has become superfluous is discharged through laughter. The same formula will also cover all cases of comic rigidity considered by Bergson, such as professional habits, fixed ideas, and modes of expression which are repeated on every occasion. All these cases aim to compare the expenditure of expectation with what is commonly required for the understanding, whereby the greater expectation depends on observation of individual variety and human plasticity. Hence in imitation the source of comic pleasure is not the comic of situation but that of expectation.

As we trace the comic pleasure in general to comparison, it is incumbent upon us to investigate also the comic element of the comparison itself, which likewise serves as a means of producing the comic. Our interest in this question will be enhanced when we recall that in the case of comparison the "feeling" as to whether something was to be classed as witty or merely comical often left us in the lurch (v. p. 114).

The subject really deserves more attention than we can bestow upon it. The main quality for which we ask in comparison is whether it is pertinent, that is, whether it really calls our attention to an existing agreement between two different objects. The original pleasure in refinding the same thing (Groos, p. 103) is not the only motive which favors the use of comparison. Besides this there is the fact that comparison is capable of a utilization which facilitates intellectual work; when for example, as is usually the case, one compares the less familiar to the more familiar, the abstract to the concrete, and explains through this comparison the more strange and the more difficult objects. With every such comparison, especially of the abstract to the concrete, there is a certain degradation and a certain economy in abstraction expenditure (in the sense of a conceptual mimicry) yet this naturally does not suffice to render prominent the character of the comic. The latter does not

emerge suddenly from the freed pleasure of
the comparison but comes gradually; there
are many cases which only touch the comic, in
which one might doubt whether they show the
comic character. The comparison undoubtedly
becomes comical when the *niveau* difference
of the expenditure of abstraction between the
two things compared becomes increased, if
something serious and strange, especially of
intellectual or moral nature is compared to
something banal and lowly. The former release of pleasure and the contribution from
the conditions of conceptual mimicry may perhaps explain the gradual change—which is determined by quantitative relations,—from the
universally pleasurable to the comic, which
takes place during the comparison. I am
certainly avoiding misunderstandings in that
I emphasize that I deduce the comic pleasure
in the comparison, not from the contrast of
the two things compared but from the difference of the two abstraction expenditures.
The strange which is difficult to grasp, the abstract and really intellectually sublime, through
its alleged agreement with a familiar lowly
one, in the imagination of which every abstraction expenditure disappears, is now itself un-
masked as something equally lowly. The

comic of comparison thus becomes reduced to a case of degradation.

The comparison, as we have seen above, can now be witty without a trace of comic admixture, especially when it happens to evade the degradation. Thus the comparison of Truth to a torch which one cannot carry through a crowd without singeing somebody's beard is pure wit, because it takes an obsolete expression (" The torch of truth ") at its full value and not at all in a comical sense, and because the torch as an object does not lack a certain distinction, though it is a concrete object. However, a comparison may just as well be witty as comic, and what is more one may be independent of the other, in that the comparison becomes an aid for certain techniques of wit, as, for example, unification or allusion. Thus Nestroy's comparison of memory to a " Warehouse " (p. 120) is simultaneously comical and witty, first, on account of the extraordinary degradation to which the psychological conception must consent in the comparison to a " Warehouse," and secondly, because he who utilizes the comparison is a clerk, and in this comparison he establishes a rather unexpected unification between psychology and his vocation. Heine's verse, " until at last the buttons tore from the pants of my patience," seems at first an excellent example of a comic degrading comparison, but on closer reflection we must ascribe to it also the attribute of wittiness, since the comparison as a means of allusion strikes into the realm of the obscene and causes a release of pleasure from the obscene. Through a union not altogether incidental the same material also gives us a resultant pleasure which is at the same time comical and witty; it does not matter whether or not the conditions of the one promote the origin of the other, such a union acts confusingly on the " feeling " whose function it is to announce to us whether we have before us wit or the comic, and only a careful examination independent of the disposition of pleasure can decide the question.

As tempting as it would be to trace these more intimate determinations of comic pleasure, the author must remember that neither his previous education nor his daily vocation justifies him in extending his investigations beyond the spheres of wit, and he must confess that it is precisely the subject of comic comparison which makes him feel his incompetence.

We are quite willing to be reminded that many authors do not recognize the clear notional and objective distinction between wit and comic, as we were impelled to do, and that they classify wit merely as "the comic of speech" or "of words." To test this view let us select one example of intentional and one of involuntary comic of speech and compare it with wit. We have already mentioned before that we are in a good position to distinguish comic from witty speech. "With a fork and with effort, his mother pulled him out of the mess," is only comical, but Heine's verse about the four castes of the population of Göttingen: "Professors, students, Philistines, and cattle," is exquisitely witty.

As an example of the intentional comic of speech I will take as a model Stettenheim's *Wippchen.* We call Stettenheim witty because he possesses the cleverness that evokes the comic. The wit which one "has" in contradistinction to the wit which one "makes," is indeed correctly conditioned by this ability. It is true that the letters of Wippchen are also witty in so far as they are interspersed with a rich collection of all sorts of witticisms, some of which very successful ones, (as "festively undressed" when he speaks of a parade of savages), but what lends the peculiar character to these productions is not these isolated witticisms, but the superabundant flow of comic speech contained therein. Originally *Wippchen* was certainly meant to represent

a satirical character, a modification of Frey-
tag's Schmock, one of those uneducated persons who trade in the educational treasure of
the nation and abuse it; but the pleasure in
the comic effect experienced in representing
this person seems gradually to have pushed to
the background the author's satirical tendency.
Wippchen's productions are for the most part
" comic nonsense." The author has justly
utilized the pleasant mood resulting from the
accumulation of such achievements to present
beside the altogether admissible material all
sorts of absurdities which would be intolerable
in themselves. Wippchen's nonsense appears
to be of a specific nature only on account of
its special technique. If we look closer into
some of these " witticisms," we find that some
forms which have impressed their character on
the whole production are especially conspicuous. Wippchen makes use mostly of compositions (fusions), of modifications of familiar
expressions and quotations. He replaces some
of the banal elements in these expressions by
others which are usually more pretentious and
more valuable. This naturally comes near to
the techniques of wit.

The Comic of Speech

Some of the fusions taken from the preface and the first pages are the following: "*Turkey's money is like the hay of the sea.*" This is only a condensation of the two expressions, " Money like hay," " Money like the sands of the sea." Or: "*I am nothing but a leafless pillar which tells of a vanished splendor,*" which is a fusion of " leafless trunk " and " a pillar which, etc." Or: "*Where is Ariadne's thread which leads out of the Scylla of this Augean stable?*" for which three different Greek myths contribute an element each.

The modifications and substitutions can be treated collectively without much forcing; their character can be seen from the following examples which are peculiar to Wippchen, they are regularly permeated by a different wording which is more fluent, most banal, and reduced to mere platitudes.

"*To hang my paper and ink high.*" The saying: " To hang one's bread-basket high," expresses metaphorically the idea of placing one under difficult conditions. But why not stretch this figure to other material?

"*Already in my youth Pegasus was alive in me.*" When the word " pegasus " is replaced by " the poet," one can recognize it as an expression often used in autobiographies. Naturally " pegasus " is not the proper word to replace the words " the poet," but it has thought associations to it and is a high-sounding word.

From Wippchen's other numerous productions some examples can be shown which present the pure comic. As an example of comic disillusionment the following can be cited: "*For hours the battle raged, finally it remained undecisive*"; an example of comical unmasking (of ignorance) is the following: "*Clio, the Medusa of history,*" or quotations like the following: "*Habent sua fata morgana.*" But our interest is aroused more by the fusions and modifications because they recall familiar techniques of wit. We may compare them to such modification witticisms as the following: "He has a great future behind him," and Lichtenberg's modification witticisms such as: "New baths heal well," etc. Should Wippchen's productions having the same technique be called witticisms, or what distinguishes them from the latter?

It is surely not difficult to answer this. Let us remember that wit presents to the hearer a double face, and forces him to two different views. In nonsense-witticisms such as those mentioned last, one view, which considers only the wording, states that they are nonsense; the other view, which, in obedience to suggestion, follows the road that leads through the hearer's unconscious, finds very good sense in these witticisms. In Wippchen's wit-like productions one of these views of wit is empty, as if stunted. It is a Janus head with only one countenance developed. One would get nowhere should he be tempted to proceed by means of this technique to the unconscious. The condensations lead to no case in which the two fused elements really result in a new sense; they fall to pieces when an attempt is made to analyze them. As in wit, the modifications and substitutions lead to a current and familiar wording, but they themselves tell us little else and as a rule nothing that is of any possible use. Hence the only thing remaining to these "witticisms" is the nonsense view. Whether such productions, which have freed themselves from one of the most essential characters of wit, should be called "bad" wit or not wit at all, every one must decide as he feels inclined.

There is no doubt that such stunted wit produces a comic effect for which we can account in more than one way. Either the comic originates through the uncovering of the unconscious modes of thinking in a manner similar to the cases considered above, or the wit originates by comparison with perfect wit. Nothing prevents us from assuming that we here deal with a union of both modes of origin of the comic pleasure. It is not to be denied that it is precisely the inadequate dependence on wit which here shapes the nonsense into comic nonsense.

Comic of Inadequacy

There are, of course, other quite apparent cases, in which such inadequacy produced by the comparison with wit, makes the nonsense irresistibly comic. The counterpart to wit, the riddle, can perhaps give us better examples for this than wit itself. A facetious question states: *What is this: It hangs on the wall and one can dry his hands on it? It would be a foolish riddle if the answer were: a towel. On the contrary this answer is rejected with the statement: No, it is a herring,—"But, for mercy's sake," is the objection, "a herring does not hang on the wall."—"But you can hang it there,"—"But who wants to dry his hands on a herring?"—"Well," is the soft answer, "you don't have to."* This explanation given through two typical displacements show how much this question lacks of being a real riddle, and because of this absolute insufficiency it impresses one as irresistibly comic, rather than mere nonsensical foolishness. Through such means, that is, by not restricting essential conditions, wit, riddles, and other forms, which in themselves produce no comic pleasure, can be made into sources of comic pleasure.

It is not so difficult to understand the case of the involuntary comic of speech which we can perhaps find realized with as much frequency as we like in the poems of Frederika Kempner.[1]

ANTI-VIVISECTION.

Fraternal sentiment should urge us
To champion the Guinea-pig,
For has it not a soul like ours,
Although most likely not as big?

Or a conversation between a loving couple.

THE CONTRAST.

The young wife whispers " I'm so happy,"
" And I!" chimes in her husband's voice,
" Because your virtues, dearest help-mate,
Reveal the wisdom of my choice."

[1] Sixth Ed., Berlin, 1891.

There is nothing here which makes one think of wit. Doubtless, however, it is the inadequacy of these " poetic productions," as the very extraordinary clumsiness of the expressions which recall the most commonplace or newspaper style, the ingenious poverty of thoughts, the absence of every trace of poetic manner of thinking or speaking,—it is all these inadequacies which make these poems comic. Nevertheless it is not at all self-evident that we should find Kempner's poems comical; many similar productions we merely consider very bad, we do not laugh at them but are rather vexed with them. But here it is the great disparity in our demand of a poem which impels us to the comic conception; where this difference is less, we are inclined to criticise rather than laugh. The comic effect of Kempner's poetic productions is furthermore assured by the additional circumstances of the lady author's unmistakably good intentions, and by the fact that her helpless phrases disarm our feeling of mockery and anger. We are now reminded of a problem the consideration of which we have so far postponed. The difference of expenditure is surely the main condition of the comic pleasure, but observation teaches that such difference does not always produce pleasure. What other conditions must

be added, or what disturbances must be
checked in order that pleasure should result
from the difference of expenditure? But before proceeding with the answers to these
questions we wish to verify what was said in
the conclusions of the former discussion,
namely, that the comic of speech is not synony-
mous with wit, and that wit must be something quite different from speech comic.

As we are about to attack the problem just
formulated, concerning the conditions of the
origin of comic pleasure from the difference of
expenditure, we may permit ourselves to facilitate this task so as to cause ourselves some
pleasure. To give a correct answer to this
question would amount to an exhaustive
presentation of the nature of the comic for
which we are fitted neither by ability nor authority. We shall therefore again be content to
elucidate the problem of the comic only
so far as it distinctly separates itself from
wit.

All theories of the comic were objected to
by the critics on the ground that in defining
the comic these theories overlooked the essential element of it. This can be seen from the
following theories, with their objections. The
comic depends on a contrasting idea; yes, in
so far as this contrast effects one comically and

in no other way. The feeling of the comic results from the dwindling away of an expectation; yes, if the disappointment does not prove
to be painful. There is no doubt that these
objections are justified, but they are overesti-
mated if one concludes from them that the essential characteristic mark of the comic has
hitherto escaped our conception. What depre-
ciates the general validity of these definitions
are conditions which are indispensable for the
origin of the comic pleasure, but which will be
searched in vain for the nature of comic pleasure. The rejection of the objections and the
explanations of the contradictions to the definitions of the comic will become easy for us,
only after we trace back comic pleasure to the
difference resulting from a comparison of two
expenditures. Comic pleasure and the effect
by which it is recognized—laughter, can originate only when this difference is no longer
utilizable and when it is capable of discharge.
We gain no pleasurable effect, or at most a
flighty feeling of pleasure in which the comic
does not appear, if the difference is put to
other use as soon as it is recognized. Just
as special precautions must be taken in wit,
in order to guard against making new use of
expenditure recognized as superfluous, so also
can comic pleasure originate only under rela-

tions which fulfil this latter condition. The cases in which such differences of expenditure originate in our ideational life are therefore uncommonly numerous, while the cases in which the comic originates from them is comparatively very rare.

The Conditions of Isolation of the Comic

Two observations obtrude themselves upon the observer who reviews even only superficially the origin of comic pleasure from the difference of expenditure; first, that there are cases in which the comic appears regularly and as if necessarily; and, in contrast to these cases, others in which this appearance depends on the conditions of the case and on the viewpoint of the observer; but secondly, that unusually large differences very often triumph over unfavorable conditions, so that the comic feeling originates in spite of it. In reference to the first point one may set up two classes, the inevitable comic and the accidental comic, although one will have to be prepared from the beginning to find exceptions in the first class to the inevitableness of the comic. It would be tempting to follow the conditions which are essential to each class.

What is important in the second class are

the conditions of which one may be designated
as the " isolation " of the comic case. A closer
analysis renders conspicuous relations something like the following:

a) The favorable condition for the origin
of comic pleasure is brought about by a general happy disposition in which " one is in the
mood for laughing." In happy toxic states almost everything seems comic, which probably
results from a comparison with the expenditure in normal conditions. For wit, the comic,
and all similar methods of gaining pleasure
from the psychic activities, are nothing but
ways to regain this happy state—euphoria—
from one single point, when it does not exist
as a general disposition of the psyche.

b) A similar favorable condition is produced by the expectation of the comic or by
putting one's self in the right mood for comic
pleasure. Hence when the intention to make
things comical exists and when this feeling is
shared by others, the differences required are
so slight that they probably would have been
overlooked had they been experienced in un-
premeditated occurrences. He who decides to
attend a comic lecture or a farce at the theater
is indebted to this intention for laughing over
things which in his everyday life would hardly
produce in him a comic effect. He finally

laughs at the recollection of having laughed, at
the expectation of laughing, and at the appearance of the one who is to present the comic,
even before the latter makes the attempt to
make him laugh. It is for this reason that
people admit that they are ashamed of that
which made them laugh at the theater.

c) Unfavorable conditions for the comic result from the kind of psychic activity which
may occupy the individual at the moment.
Imaginative or mental activity tending towards
serious aims disturbs the discharging capacity
of the investing energies which the activity
needs for its own displacements, so that only
unexpected and great differences of expenditure can break through to form comic pleasure. All manner of mental processes far
enough removed from the obvious to cause a
suspension of ideational mimicry are unfavorable to the comic; in abstract contemplation
there is hardly any room left for the comic,
except when this form of thinking is suddenly
interrupted.

d) The occasion for releasing comic pleasure vanishes when the attention is fixed on the
comparison capable of giving rise to the comic.
Under such circumstances the comic force is
lost from that which is otherwise sure to produce a comic effect. A movement or a mental

activity cannot become comical to him whose interest is fixed at the time of comparing this movement with a standard which distinctly presents itself to him. Thus the examiner does not see the comical in the nonsense produced by the student in his ignorance; he is simply annoyed by it, whereas the offender's classmates who are more interested in his chances of passing the examination than in what he knows, laugh heartily over the same nonsense. The teacher of dancing or gymnastics seldom has any eyes for the comic movements of his pupils, and the preacher entirely loses sight of humanity's defects of character, which the writer of comedy brings out with so much effect. The comic process cannot stand examination by the attention, it must be able to proceed absolutely unnoticed in a manner similar to wit. But for good reasons, it would contradict the nomenclature of "conscious processes" which I have used in *The Interpretation of Dreams,* if one wished to call it of necessity *unconscious.* It rather belongs to the *foreconscious,* and one may use the fitting name "automatic" for all those processes which are enacted in the foreconscious and dispense with the attention energy which is connected with consciousness. The process of comparison of the expenditures must remain automatic if it is to produce comic pleasure.

Conditions Disturbing the Discharge

e) It is exceedingly disturbing to the comic if the case from which it originates gives rise at the same time to a marked release of affect. The discharge of the affective difference is then as a rule excluded. Affects, disposition, and the attitude of the individual in occasional cases make it clear that the comic comes or goes with the viewpoint of the individual person; that only in exceptional cases is there an absolute comic. The dependence or relativity of the comic is therefore much greater than of wit, which never happens but is regularly made, and at its production one may already give attention to the conditions under which it finds acceptance. But affective development is the most intensive of the conditions which disturb the comic, the significance of which is well known.[1] It is therefore said that the comic feeling comes most in tolerably indifferent cases which evince no strong feelings or interests. Nevertheless it is just in cases with affective release that one may witness the production of a particularly strong expenditure-

[1] "You may well laugh, that no longer concerns you."

difference in the automatism of discharge.
When Colonel Butler answers Octavio's ad-
monitions with "bitter laughter," exclaiming:

"Thanks from the house of Austria!"

his bitterness has thus not prevented the laughter which results from the recollection of the
disappointment which he believes he has experienced; and on the other hand, the magnitude
of this disappointment could not have been
more impressively depicted by the poet than
by showing it capable of affecting laughter in
the midst of the storm of unchained affects.
It is my belief that this explanation may be
applicable in all cases in which laughing occurs
on other than pleasurable occasions, and in
conjunction with exceedingly painful or tense
affects.

f) If we also mention that the development
of the comic pleasure can be promoted by
means of any other pleasurable addition to the
case which acts like a sort of contact-effect
(after the manner of the fore-pleasure principle in the tendency-wit), then we have discussed surely not all the conditions of comic
pleasure, yet enough of them to serve our purpose. We then see that no other assumption
so easily covers these conditions, as well as the
inconstancy and dependence of the comic ef-

fect, as this: the assumption that comic pleasure is derived from the discharge of a difference, which under many conditions can be diverted to a different use than discharge.

It still remains to give a thorough consideration of the comic of the sexual and obscene, but we shall only skim over it with a few observations. Here, too, we shall take the act of exposing one's body as the starting-point. An accidental exposure produces a comical effect on us, because we compare the ease with which we attained the enjoyment of this view with the great expenditure otherwise necessary for the attainment of this object. The case thus comes nearer to the naïve-comic, but it is simpler than the latter. In every case of exhibitionism in which we are made spectators— or, in the case of the smutty joke hearers,— we play the part of the third person, and the person exposed is made comical. We have heard that it is the purpose of wit to replace obscenity and in this manner to reopen a source of comic pleasure that has been lost. On the contrary, spying out an exposure forms no example of the comic for the one spying, because the effort he exerts thereby abrogates the condition of comic pleasure; the only thing remaining is the sexual pleasure in what is seen. If the spy relates to another what he has seen, the person looked at again becomes comical, because the viewpoint that predominates is that the expenditure was omitted which would have been necessary for the concealment of the private parts. At all events, the sphere of the sexual or obscene offers the richest opportunities for gaining comic pleasure beside the pleasurable sexual stimulation, as it exposes the person's dependence on his physical needs (degradation) or it can uncover behind the spiritual love the physical demands of the same (unmasking.)

The Psychogenesis of the Comic

An invitation to seek the understanding of the comic in its psychogenesis comes surprisingly from Bergson's well written and stimulating book *Laughter*. Bergson, whose formula for the conception of the comic character has already become known to us— "mechanization of life," "the substitution of something mechanical for the natural"— reaches by obvious associations from automatism to the automaton, and seeks to trace a series of comic effects to the blurred memories of children's toys. In this connection he once reaches this viewpoint, which, to be sure, he soon drops; he seeks to trace the comic to the after-effect of childish pleasure. "Perhaps we ought even to carry simplification still farther, and, going back to our earliest recollection, try to discover in the games that amused us as children the first faint traces of the combinations that make us laugh as grown-up persons." . . . "Above all, we are too apt to ignore the childish element, so to speak, latent in most of our joyful emotions" (p. 67). As we have now traced wit to that childish playing with words and thoughts which is prohibited by the rational critic, we must be tempted to trace also these infantile roots of the comic, conjectured by Bergson.

As a matter of fact we meet a whole series of conditions which seem most promising, when we examine the relation of the comic to the child. The child itself does not by any means seem comic to us, although its character fulfills all conditions which, in comparison to our own, would result in a comic difference. Thus we see the immoderate expenditure of motion as well as the slight psychic expenditure, the control of the psychic activities through bodily functions, and other features. The child gives us a comic impression only when it does not behave as a child but as an earnest grown-up, and even then it affects us only in the same

manner as other persons in disguise; but as
long as it retains the nature of the child our
perception of it furnishes us a pure pleasure,
which perhaps recalls the comic. We call it
naïve in so far as it displays to us the absence
of inhibitions, and we call naïve-comic those of
its utterances which in another we would have
considered obscene or witty.

On the other hand the child lacks all feeling for the comic. This sentence seems to say
no more than that this comic feeling, like many
others, first makes its appearance in the course
of psychic development; and that would by no
means be remarkable, especially since we must
admit that it shows itself distinctly even during years which must be accredited to childhood. Nevertheless it can be demonstrated
that the assertion that the child lacks feeling
for the comic has a deeper meaning than one
would suppose. In the first place it will readily be seen that it cannot be different, if our
conception is correct, that the comic feeling results from a difference of expenditure produced in the effort to understand the other.
Let us again take comic motion as an example.
The comparison which furnishes the difference
reads as follows, when put in conscious formulæ: " So he does it," and: " So I would do
it," or " So I have done it." But the child

lacks the standard contained in the second
sentence, it understands simply through imitation; it just does it. Education of the child
furnishes it with the standard: "So you shall
do it," and if it now makes use of the same
in comparisons, the nearest conclusion is: "He
has not done it right, and I can do it better."
In this case it laughs at the other, it laughs
at him with a feeling of superiority. There
is nothing to prevent us from tracing this
laughter also to a difference of expenditure;
but according to the analogy with the examples of laughter occurring in us we may conclude that the comic feeling is not experienced
by the child when it laughs as an expression
of superiority. It is a laughter of pure pleasure. In our own case whenever the judgment
of our own superiority occurs we smile rather
than laugh, or if we laugh, we are still able
to distinguish clearly this conscious realization
of our superiority from the comic which makes
us laugh.

It is probably correct to say that in many
cases which we perceive as "comical" and
which we cannot explain, the child laughs out
of pure pleasure, whereas the child's motives
are clear and assignable. If for instance,
some one slips on the street and falls, we laugh
because this impression—we know not why—

is comical. The child laughs in the same case out of a feeling of superiority or out of joy over the calamity of others. It amounts to saying: "You fell, but I did not." Certain pleasure motives of the child seems to be lost for us grown-ups, but as a substitute for these we perceive under the same conditions the "comic" feeling.

The Infantile and the Comic

If we were permitted to generalize, it would seem very tempting to transfer the desired specific character of the comic into the awakening of the infantile, and to conceive the comic as a regaining of "lost infantile laughing." One could then say, "I laugh every time over a difference of expenditure between the other and myself, when I discover in the other the child." Or expressed more precisely, the whole comparison leading to the comic would read as follows:

"He does it this way—I do it differently—
He does it just as I did when I was a child."

This laughter would thus result every time from the comparison between the ego of the grown-up and the ego of the child. The uncertainty itself of the comic difference, causing now the lesser and now the greater expenditure to appear comical to me, would correspond to the infantile determination; the comic therein is actually always on the side of the infantile.

This is not contradicted by the fact that the child itself as an object of comparison does not make a comic impression on me but a purely pleasurable one, nor by the fact that this comparison with the infantile produces a comic effect only when any other use of the difference is avoided. For the conditions of the discharge come thereby into consideration. Everything that confines a psychic process in an association of ideas works against the discharge of the surplus occupation of energy and directs the same to other utilization; whatever isolates a psychic act favors the discharge. By consciously focussing on the child as the person of comparison, the discharge necessary for the production of comic pleasure therefore becomes impossible; only in foreconscious energetic states is there a similar approach to the isolation which we may moreover also ascribe to the psychic processes in the child. The addition to the comparison: "Thus I have also done it as a child," from which the comic effect would emanate, could come into consideration for the average difference only when no other association could obtain control over the freed surplus.

If we still continue with our attempt to find the nature of the comic in the foreconscious association of the infantile, we have to go a step further than Bergson and admit that the comparison resulting in the comic need not necessarily awake old childish pleasure and play, but that it is enough if it touches the childish nature in general, perhaps even childish pain. Herein we deviate from Bergson, but remain consistent with ourselves, when we connect the comic pleasure not with remembered pleasure but always with a comparison. This is possible, for cases of the first kind comprise in a measure those which are regularly and irresistibly comic. Let us now draw up the scheme of the comic possibilities instanced above. We stated that the comic difference would be found either

(a) through a comparison between the other and one's self, or (b) through a comparison altogether within the other, or (c) through a comparison altogether within one's self.

In the first case the other would appear to me as a child, in the second he would put himself on the level of a child, and in the third I would find the child in myself. To the first class belong the comic of movement and of forms, of psychic activity and of character. The infantile corresponding to it would be the motion-impulse and the inferior mental and moral development of the child, so that the fool would perhaps become comical to me by reminding me of a lazy child, and the bad person by reminding me of a naughty child. The only time one might speak of a childish pleasure lost to grown-ups would be where the child's own motion pleasure came into consideration.

The second case, in which the comic altogether depends on identification with the other, comprises numerous possibilities such as the comic situation, exaggeration (caricature), imitation, degradation, and unmasking. It is under this head that the presentation of infantile viewpoints mostly take place. For the comic situation is largely based on embarrassment, in which we feel again the helplessness of the child. The worst of these embarrassments, the disturbance of other activities through the imperative demands of natural wants, corresponds to the child's lack of control of the physical functions. Where the comic situation acts through repetitions it is based on the pleasure of constant repetition peculiar to the child (asking questions, telling stories), through which it makes itself a nuisance to grown-ups. Exaggeration, which also affords pleasure even to the grown-up in so far as it is justified by his reason, corresponds to the characteristic want of moderation in the child, and its ignorance of all quantitative relations which it later really learns to know as qualitative. To keep within bounds, to practice moderation even in permissible feelings is a late fruit of education, and is gained through opposing inhibitions of the psychic activity acquired in the same association. Wherever this association is weakened as in the unconscious of dreams and in the monoideation of the psychoneuroses, the want of moderation of the child again makes its appearance.

The understanding of comic imitation has caused us many difficulties so long as we left out of consideration the infantile factor. But imitation is the child's best art and is the impelling motive of most of its playing. The child's ambition is not so much to distinguish himself among his equals as to imitate the big fellows. The relation of the child to the grown-up determines also the comic of degradation, which corresponds to the lowering of the grown-up in the life of the child. Few things can afford the child greater pleasure than when the grown-up lowers himself to its level, disregards his superiority, and plays with the child as its equal. The alleviation which furnishes the child pure pleasure is a debasement used by the adult as a means of making things comic and as a source of comic pleasure. As for unmasking we know that it is based on degradation.

The infantile determination of the third case, the comic of expectation, presents most of the difficulties; this really explains why those authors who put this case to the foreground in their conception of the comic, found no occasion to consider the infantile factor in their studies of the comic. The comic of expectation is farthest from the child's thoughts, the ability to understand this is the latest quality to appear in him. Most of those cases which produce a comic effect in the grown-up are probably felt by the child as a disappointment. One can refer, however, to the blissful expectation and gullibility of the child in order to understand why one considers himself as comical "as a child," when he succumbs to comic disappointment.

If the preceding remarks produce a certain probability that the comic feeling may be translated into the thought; everything is comic that does not fit the grown-up, I still do not feel bold enough,—in view of my whole position to the problem of the comic—to defend this last proposition with the same earnestness as those that I formulated before. I am unable to decide whether the lowering to the level of the child is only a special case of comic degradation, or whether everything comical fundamentally depends on the degradation to the level of the child.[1]

Humor

An examination of the comic, however superficial it may be, would be most incomplete if it did not devote at least a few remarks to the consideration of *humor*. There is so little doubt as to the essential relationship between the two that a tentative explanation of the comic must furnish at least one component for the understanding of humor. It does not matter how much appropriate and important material was presented as an appreciation of humor, which, as one of the highest psychic functions, enjoys the special favor of thinkers, we still cannot elude the temptation to express its essence through an approach to the formulæ given for wit and the comic.

[1] That comic pleasure has its source in the "quantitative contrast," in the comparison of big and small, which ultimately also expresses the essential relation of the child to the grown-up, would indeed be a peculiar coincidence if the comic had nothing else to do with the infantile.

We have heard that the release of painful emotions is the strongest hindrance to the comic effect. Just as aimless motion causes harm, stupidity mischief, and disappointment pain;—the possibility of a comic effect eventually ends, at least for him who cannot defend himself against such pain, who is himself affected by it or must participate in it, whereas the disinterested party shows by his behavior that the situation of the case in question contains everything necessary to produce a comic effect. Humor is thus a means to gain pleasure despite the painful affects which disturb it; it acts as a substitute for this affective development, and takes its place. If we are in a situation which tempts us to liberate painful affects according to our habits, and motives then urge us to suppress these affects *statu nascendi,* we have the conditions for humor. In the cases just cited the person affected by misfortune, pain, etc., could obtain humoristic pleasure while the disinterested party laughs over the comic pleasure. We can only say that the pleasure of humor results at the cost of this discontinued liberation of affect; it originates through the *economized expenditure of affect.*

The Economy in Expenditure of Affect

Humor is the most self-sufficient of the forms of the comic; its process consummating itself in one single person and the participation of another adds nothing new to it. I can enjoy the pleasure of humor originating in myself without feeling the necessity of imparting it to another. It is not easy to tell what happens during the production of humoristic pleasure in a person; but one gains a certain insight by investigating these cases of humor which have emanated from persons with whom we have entered into a sympathetic understanding. By sympathetically understanding the humoristic person in these cases one gets the same pleasure. The coarsest form of humor, the so-called humor of the gallows or grim-humor (*Galgenhumor*), may enlighten us in this regard. The rogue, on being led to execution on Monday, remarked: "Yes, this week is beginning well." This is really a witticism, as the remark is quite appropriate in itself, on the other hand it is displaced in the most nonsensical fashion, as there can be no further happening for him this week. But it required humor to make such wit, that is, to overlook what distinguished the beginning of this week from other weeks, and to deny the difference which could give rise to motives for very particular emotional feelings. The case is the same when on the way to the gallows he requests a neckerchief for his bare neck, in order to guard against taking cold, a precaution which would be quite praiseworthy under different circumstances, but becomes exceedingly superfluous and indifferent in view of the impending fate of this same neck. We must say that there is something like greatness of soul in this *blague,* in this clinging to his usual nature and in deviating from that which would overthrow and drive this nature into despair. This form of grandeur of humor thus appears unmistakably in cases in which our admiration is not inhibited by the circumstances of the humoristic person.

In Victor Hugo's *Ernani* the bandit who entered into a conspiracy against his king, Charles I, of Spain, (Charles V, as the German Emperor), falls into the hands of his most powerful enemy; he foresees his fate; as one convicted of high treason his head will fall. But this prospect does not deter him from introducing himself as a hereditary Grandee of Spain and from declaring that he has no intention of waiving any prerogative belonging to such personage. A Grandee of

Spain could appear before his royal master with his head covered. Well:

> " Nos têtes ont le droit
> De tomber couvertes devant de toi." [1]

This is excellent humor and if we do not laugh on hearing it, it is because our admiration covers the humoristic pleasure. In the case of the rogue who did not wish to take cold on the way to the gallows we roar with laughter. The situation which should have driven this criminal to despair, might have evoked in us int ..se pity, but this pity is inhibited because we understand that he who is most concerned is quite indifferent to the situation. As a result of this understanding the expenditure for pity, which was already prepared in us, became inapplicable and we laughed it off. The indifference of the rogue, which we notice has cost him a great expenditure of psychic labor, infects us as it were.

Economy of sympathy is one of the most frequent sources of humoristic pleasure. Mark Twain's humor usually follows this mechanism. When he tells us about the life of his brother, how, as an employee in a large road-building enterprise, he was hurled into the air through a premature explosion of a

[1] " Our heads have the right to fall covered before thee."

blast, to come to earth again far from the place where he was working, feelings of sympathy for this unfortunate are invariably aroused in us. We should like to inquire whether he sustained no injury in this accident; but the continuation of the story that the brother lost a half-day's pay for being away from the place he worked diverts us entirely from sympathy and makes us almost as hard-hearted as that employer, and just as indifferent to the possible injury to the victim's health. Another time Mark Twain presents us his pedigree, which he traces back almost as far back as one of the companions of Columbus. But after describing the character of this ancestor, whose entire possessions consisted of several pieces of linen each bearing a different mark, we cannot help laughing at the expense of the stored-up piety, a piety which characterized our frame of mind at the beginning of this family history. The mechanism of humoristic pleasure is not disturbed by our knowing that this family history is a fictitious one, and that this fiction serves a satirical tendency to expose the embellishments which result in imparting such pedigrees to others; it is just as independent of the conditions of reality as the manufactured comic. Another of Mark Twain's stories relates how his brother constructed for himself subter-

ranean quarters into which he brought a bed, a
table, and a lamp, and that as a roof he used
a large piece of sail-cloth with a hole through
the centre; how during the night after the
room was completed, a cow being driven home
fell through the opening in the ceiling on to
the table and extinguished the lamp; how his
brother helped patiently to hoist the animal out
and to rearrange everything; how he did the
same thing when the same disturbance was repeated the following night; and then every
succeeding night; such a story becomes comical through repetition. But Mark Twain
closes with the information that in the forty-
sixth night when the cow again fell through,
his brother finally remarked that the thing was
beginning to grow monotonous; and here we
can no longer restrain our humoristic pleasure,
for we had long expected to hear how the
brother would express his anger over this
chronic *malheur*. The slight humor which we
draw from our own life we usually produce at
the expense of anger instead of irritating ourselves.[1]

---

[1] The excellent humoristic effect of a character like that of
the fat knight, Sir John Falstaff, is based on economized contempt and indignation. To be sure we recognize in him the
unworthy glutton and fashionably dressed swindler, but our condemnation is disarmed through a whole series of factors. We
understand that he knows himself to be just as we estimate him;

Forms of Humor

The forms of humor are extraordinarily varied according to the nature of the emotional feelings which are economized in favor of humor, as sympathy, anger, pain, compassion,

he impresses us through his wit; and besides that, his physical deformity produces a contact-effect in favor of a comic conception of his personality instead of a serious one; as if our demands for morality and honor must recoil from such a big stomach. His activities are altogether harmless and are almost excused by the comic lowness of those he deceives. We admit that the poor devil has a right to live and enjoy himself like any one else, and we almost pity him because in the principal situation we find him a puppet in the hands of one much his superior. It is for this reason that we cannot bear him any grudge and turn all we economize in him in indignation into comic pleasure which he otherwise provides. Sir John's own humor really emanates from the superiority of an ego which neither his physical nor his moral defects can rob of its joviality and security.

On the other hand the courageous knight Don Quixote de la Mancha is a figure who possesses no humor, and in his seriousness furnishes us a pleasure which can be called humoristic although its mechanism shows a decided deviation from that of humor. Originally Don Quixote is a purely comic figure, a big child whose fancies from his books on knighthood have gone to his head. It is known that at first the poet wanted to show only that phase of his character, and that the creation gradually outgrew the author's original intentions. But after the poet endowed this ludicrous person with the profoundest wisdom and noblest aims and made him the symbolic representation of an idealism, a man who believed in the realization of his aims, who took duties seriously and promises literally, he ceased to be a comic personality. Like humoristic pleasure which results from a prevention of emotional feelings it originates here through the disturbance of comic pleasure. However, in these examples we already depart perceptibly from the simple cases of humor.

etc. And this series seems incomplete because the sphere of humor experiences a constant enlargement, as often as an artist or writer succeeds in mastering humoristically the, as yet, unconquered emotional feelings and in making them, through artifices similar to those in the above example, a source of humoristic pleasure. Thus the artists of *Simplicissimus* have worked wonders in gaining humor at the expense of fear and disgust. The manifestations of humor are above all determined by two peculiarities, which are connected with the conditions of its origin. In the first place, humor may appear fused with wit or any other form of the comic; whereby it is entrusted with the task of removing a possible emotional development which would form a hindrance to the pleasurable effect. Secondly, it can entirely set aside this emotional development or only partially, which is really the more frequent case, because the simpler function and the different forms of "broken"[1] humor, results in that humor which smiles under its tears. It withdraws from the affect a part of its energy and gives instead the accompanying humoristic sound.

As may be noticed by former examples the

---

[1] A term which is used in quite a different sense in the *Aesthetik* of Theo. Vischer.

humoristic pleasure gained by entering into sympathy with a thing results from a special technique resembling displacement through which the liberation of affect held ready is disappointed and the energy occupation is deflected to other, and, not often, to secondary matters. This does not help us, however, to understand the process by which the displacement from the development of affect proceeds in the humoristic person himself. We see that the recipient intimates the producer of the humor in his psychic processes, but we discover nothing thereby concerning the forces which make this process possible in the latter.

We can only say, when, for example, somebody succeeds in paying no heed to a painful affect because he holds before himself the greatness of the world's interest as a contrast to his own smallness, that we see in this no function of humor but one of philosophic thinking, and we gain no pleasure even if we put ourselves into his train of thought. The humoristic displacement is therefore just as impossible in the light of conscious attention as is the comic comparison; like the latter it is connected with the condition to remain in the foreconscious—that is to say, to remain automatic.

One reaches some solution of humoristic displacement if one examines it in the light of a
defense process. The defense processes are
the psychic correlates of the flight reflex and
follow the task of guarding against the origin
of pain from inner sources; in fulfilling this
task they serve the psychic function as an
automatic adjustment, which finally proves
harmful and therefore must be subjected .to
the control of the conscious thinking. A
definite form of this defense, the failure of repression, I have demonstrated as the effective
mechanism in the origin of the psychoneuroses.
Humor can now be conceived as the loftiest
variant of this defense activity. It disdains to
withdraw from conscious attention the ideas
which are connected with the painful affect, as
repression does, and thus it overcomes the defense automatism. It brings this about by
finding the means to withdraw the energy resulting from the liberation of pain which is held
in readiness and through discharge changes the
same into pleasure. It is even credible that it is
again the connection with the infantile that
puts at humor's disposal the means for this
function. Only in childhood did we experience
intensively painful affects over which to-day as
grown-ups we would laugh; just as a humorist
laughs over his present painful affects. The

elevation of his ego, of which humoristic displacement gives evidence,—the translation of
which would read: I am too big to have these
causes affect me painfully—he could find in
the comparison of his present ego with his infantile ego. This conception is to some extent
confirmed by the rôle which falls to the infantile in the neurotic processes of repression.

The Relation of Humor to Wit and Comic

On the whole humor is closer to the comic
than wit. Like the former its psychic localization is in the foreconscious, whereas wit,
as we had to assume, is formed as a compromise between the unconscious and the foreçon-
scious. On the other hand, humor has no share
in the peculiar nature in which wit and the
comic meet, a peculiarity which perhaps we have
not hitherto emphasized strongly enough. It
is a condition for the origin of the comic that
we be induced to apply—either *simultaneously*
or in rapid succession—to the same thought
function two different modes of ideas, between
which the " comparison " then takes place and
thus forms the comic difference. Such differences originate between the expenditure of the
stranger and one's own, between the usual expenditure and the emergency expenditure, be-

tween an anticipated expenditure and one which has already occurred.[1]

The difference between two forms of conception resulting simultaneously, which work with different expenditures, comes into consideration in wit, in respect to the hearer. The one of these two conceptions, by taking the hints contained in the witticism, follows the train of thought through the unconscious, while the other conception remains on the surface and presents the witticism like any wording from the foreconscious which has become conscious. Perhaps it would not be considered an unjustified statement if we should refer the pleasure of the witticism heard to the difference between these two forms of presentation.

Concerning wit we here repeat our former statement concerning its Janus-like doublefacedness, a simile we used when the relation between wit and the comic still appeared to us unsettled.[2]

[1] If one does not hesitate to do some violence to the conception of expectation, one may ascribe—according to the process of Lipps—a very large sphere of the comic to the comic of expectation; but probably the most original cases of the comic which result through a comparison of a strange expenditure with one's own will fit least into this conception.

[2] The characteristic of the "double face" naturally did not escape the authors. Melinaud, from whom I borrowed the above expression, conceives the condition for laughing in the following formula: "Ce qui fait rire c'est qui est à la fois, d'un coté, absurde et de l'autre, familier" ("Pourquoi rit-on?" *Revue de*

The character thus put into the foreground becomes indistinct when we deal with humor. To be sure, we feel the humoristic pleasure where an emotional feeling is evaded, which we might have expected as a pleasure usually belonging to the situation; and in so far humor really falls under the broadened conception of the comic of expectation. But in humor it is no longer a question of two different kinds of presentations having the same content; the fact that the situation comes under the domination of a painful emotional feeling which should have been avoided, puts an end to possible comparison with the nature in the comic and in wit. The humoristic displacement is really a case of that different kind of utilization of a freed expenditure which proved to be so dangerous for the comic effect.

Formulæ for Wit, Comic, and Humor

Now, that we have reduced the mechanism of humoristic pleasure to a formula analogous

deux mondes, February, 1895). This formula fits in better with wit than with the comic, but it really does not altogether cover the former. Bergson (l. c., p. 96) defines the comic situation by the "reciprocal interference of series," and states: "A situation is invariably comic when it belongs simultaneously to two altogether independent series of events and is capable of being interpreted in two entirely different meanings at the same time." According to Lipps the comic is "the greatness and smallness of the same."

to the formula of comic pleasure and of wit, we are at the end of our task. It has seemed to us that the pleasure of wit originates from an *economy of expenditure in inhibition,* of the comic from an *economy of expenditure in thought,* and of humor from an *economy of expenditure in feeling.* All three activities of our psychic apparatus derive pleasure from economy. They all strive to bring back from the psychic activity a pleasure which has really been lost in the development of this activity. For the euphoria which we are thus striving to obtain is nothing but the state of a bygone time in which we were wont to defray our psychic work with slight expenditure. It is the state of our childhood in which we did not know the comic, were incapable of wit, and did not need humor to make us happy.

INDEX